# Therapeutic Precision: In-Depth Guide to Dosage Calculation in Medical Settings

## Methodologies, Common Errors, Technological Tools, and Guidelines for Safe and Personalized Medication Administration

Florence Healingheart

# 1. Introduction

## Purpose and Importance of Dosage Calculators for Nursing

The art and science of nursing demand competence and precision, especially when it comes to administering medications to patients. Every day, nurses around the world in clinics and hospitals are responsible for the safe and accurate intake of medicines by patients. To ensure this, understanding and proficiency in dosage calculations are essential.

A nursing dosage calculator is not just a tool that simplifies a mathematical task. It is a safeguard that ensures patients receive the right amount of medication necessary for their treatment, preventing overdose or underdose. These calculators take into account the patient's specific needs, such as age, weight, and condition, and help translate this information into a safe and effective drug dosage.

## The Need for Precision in the Clinical World

In the field of healthcare, error is not just a simple oversight; it can have serious, potentially fatal consequences. This is especially true when it comes to medication dosing. A calculation error could lead to an overdose, which could cause an adverse reaction or, in the worst-case scenario, death. Conversely, underdosing could render a treatment ineffective, compromising a patient's recovery or prolonging their suffering.

In a clinical scenario, every decision and action must be executed with the utmost care and accuracy. Precision is not just a desirable skill but an absolute necessity. In the context of medication administration, precision ensures that each patient receives the right amount of medication based on their unique needs, maximizing the benefits of treatment and minimizing risks.

Continual education and the acquisition of skills necessary for accurately calculating dosages are essential for every nurse. Through practice and training, nurses can ensure they provide the best and safest care possible to their patients.

With this book, we are committed to providing a comprehensive and practical guide to understanding and mastering dosage calculations in various clinical scenarios. Through examples, exercises, and clear explanations, we hope to make this crucial task a bit less intimidating and much more accessible.

## The Deep Connection Between Nursing and Dosage Calculation

At the heart of nursing is a profound and unwavering commitment to the well-being of patients. Nurses, day after day, dedicate themselves to providing compassionate, high-quality care based on specialized skills and a broad knowledge base. One of the fundamental skills every nurse must possess is the ability to accurately calculate medication dosages.

The act of administering a medication, while seeming simple on the surface, is actually a complex process that requires attention to detail and precision. When a physician prescribes a medication, the dose is often based on various factors, including the patient's weight, age, clinical condition, and even the pharmacokinetics and pharmacodynamics of the drug itself. However, this prescription must then be translated into a concrete action by the nurse, who must prepare and administer the medication.

In this context, dosage calculation is not a simple mathematical exercise. It is rather a critical set of decisions that must be made with care to ensure patient safety. Every medication has a therapeutic profile, representing the range of doses within which it is both safe and effective. Going beyond this range could lead to toxic effects, while staying below it may not provide the desired therapeutic benefit.

Furthermore, in a fast-paced clinical environment where patients often have multiple comorbidities and are on multiple medications, the management and safe administration of drugs become even more complex. There are pharmacological interactions to consider, as well as potential adverse reactions. Additionally, patients may have renal or hepatic insufficiencies that alter drug metabolism and, as a result, require dosage adjustments.

This is why dosage calculation is much more than a formula; it is the synthesis of anatomy, physiology, pharmacology, and mathematics. It requires a deep understanding not only of the drug in question but also of the patient as an individual.

In daily practice, nurses often find themselves having to make quick but critical calculations. For example, in an emergency situation where every second counts, the ability to calculate a dosage quickly can make the difference between life and death. At the same time, in a palliative care context where patient comfort is of primary importance, the ability to administer the right dose of an analgesic can have a profound impact on the patient's quality of life.

It is interesting to note that, despite the increasing digitization of medicine and the availability of advanced tools and technologies, competence in dosage calculations remains fundamental. While technologies can assist and support, the final decision always rests with the nurse. And in this decision, training, competence, and experience play a crucial role. Therefore, dosage calculation represents an intersection of science and art in nursing. While science provides the tools and knowledge to make accurate calculations, it is the art of nursing, with its attention to the patient as an individual and its dedication to well-being, that guides the application of this knowledge in practice. Finally, it is essential to recognize that, while dosage calculation is a technical skill, it has a profoundly human impact. Every calculation, every decision, involves a person with a history, a family, hopes, and fears. This intersection of science, art, and humanity makes dosage calculation one of the most vital and precious skills in nursing. And through continuous education and practice, nurses can ensure they exercise this skill with the utmost care and integrity.

The role of the nurse, in every facet, embodies a combination of knowledge, empathy, and technical ability. In few other professional fields, a single technical decision has such an immediate impact on an individual's life and well-being. Dosage calculation, although it may seem like a mere mathematical application, is actually an act of care deeply rooted in the central mission of nursing. Every single dose administered is the result of a series of assessments and decisions. Not only is the physician's prescription considered, but also the expected physiological response of the patient, potential pharmacological interactions, and the patient's ever-evolving clinical conditions. For instance, the same dose of a medication might have different effects on a healthy patient compared to a patient with renal insufficiency. These nuances, which go beyond the mere dosage formula, are what nurses navigate every day. Another aspect to consider is the very environment in which nurses work. In a high-pressure hospital setting, where every minute counts, the ability to quickly and accurately perform dosage calculations is essential. It's not just about speed, but also about resisting distractions and maintaining focus amid chaos, noise, and constant interruptions. Furthermore, there are moments when a nurse may need to rely on clinical judgment, based on experience and intuition, as well as pure numbers. Imagine, for instance, having a pediatric patient showing signs of distress, but whose exact weight is not known. While an accurate dosage calculation based on weight would be ideal, the nurse may need to make an informed estimate based on observation and experience to administer vital medication. The ethical implications of dosage calculation are equally profound. The nursing profession is guided by an ethical code that emphasizes the dignity, worth, and unique rights of every individual. Every decision regarding medication dosage must reflect these ethical priorities. Providing safe, effective, and appropriate care is at the core of this ethical commitment. Then there's the relational dimension of nursing, which intertwines with dosage calculation. The nurse not only administers medications but often also serves as an educator, counselor, and supporter. The patient or their family may have questions or concerns about a medication, its dosage, or its side effects. The nurse must be prepared not only to calculate and administer the correct dosage but also to effectively communicate medication-related information, address concerns, and help the patient and their family understand its importance and benefits. Additionally, lifelong learning and continuous education are essential aspects of the nursing profession. Pharmacology is a constantly evolving science, with new drugs and therapies emerging regularly. Nurses must be proactive in updating their skills and knowledge, ensuring they are always up to date with current best practices in dosage and medication administration. Throughout all of this, dosage calculation remains a focal point, a daily ritual symbolizing the nurse's commitment to providing safe, compassionate, and effective care. Through every digit, formula, and decision, the nurse's deep responsibility for the lives and well-being of patients is reflected. And this responsibility, though burdensome, is also a privilege, as it offers nurses the opportunity to make a difference in people's lives every single day. The precision in dosage calculation is just one part of the complex equation of healthcare. Behind every administered dose is a profound network of knowledge that intertwines with the nurse's experience, training, and intuition. This calculation transcends mere mathematics and becomes an exercise in clinical competence and professional judgment.

While errors in dosage can have serious consequences for a patient's health, the ability to calculate dosages accurately is closely linked to the patient's trust in the healthcare system and their care team. This trust is essential for building an effective therapeutic relationship. When a patient feels confident that the care they receive is accurate and personalized, they are more likely to adhere to medical recommendations, communicate openly with their care team, and actively participate in their healing and well-being. The evolution of technology has brought new challenges and opportunities in the field of dosage calculation. While technological devices can assist and, in some cases, automate the calculation process, the ultimate responsibility always remains with the human overseeing and authorizing the administration. Technology can help reduce errors, but human competence, judgment, and attention to detail are irreplaceable. The challenges nurses face in dosage calculation are not static. Every day, new medications enter the market, each with its specific indications, mechanisms of action, and dosage profiles. Nurses must keep their skills up-to-date, not only by learning how these new drugs work but also how they integrate into the existing therapeutic regimens of patients. In light of these challenges, the importance of interprofessional collaboration also emerges. Nurses, although often at the forefront of medication administration, are not isolated in this responsibility. They work closely with pharmacists, physicians, and other healthcare professionals to ensure that each patient receives the correct dose of the appropriate medication. This collaboration is essential because each member of the care team brings a unique and valuable perspective. Beyond interprofessional collaboration, there is also an aspect of self-reflection and self-assessment in dosage calculation. Nurses, in their commitment to professional excellence, must be able to recognize their own limits and seek help or clarification when needed. The culture of patient safety emphasizes the importance of admitting and learning from mistakes, rather than concealing them. The educational dimension is equally critical. Experienced nurses often serve as mentors to their less experienced colleagues, sharing their knowledge and providing practical guidance in the field. This transmission of knowledge is fundamental to maintaining high standards of care and ensuring that future generations of nurses are equally competent in dosage calculation. The act of calculating a dosage is not just a technical task. It is an act of care, an exercise in clinical judgment, and a manifestation of the nurse's dedication to the health and well-being of the patient. Through dosage calculation, nurses demonstrate their commitment not only to patient safety but also to the integrity of their profession. In each calculation lies the promise of the nurse to provide evidence-based, personalized, high-quality care. And this promise, supported by education, experience, and passion, is what makes the nursing profession so essential in the healthcare landscape. In conclusion, dosage calculation in nursing is not merely a mathematical task but a fundamental and multidimensional aspect of clinical practice. It goes far beyond the mere administration of medications, as it deeply intertwines with professional responsibility, ethics, education, and communication. First and foremost, every calculation is a concrete commitment to patient safety. Even a minor error can have serious repercussions on the patient's health, affecting not only their physical well-being but also the trust they place in the healthcare system. This trust, built on precise and attentive nursing practice, is essential for establishing effective therapeutic relationships, which are the foundation of quality care. The complexity of dosage calculation is amplified by the rapid evolution of pharmacology and the increasing diversity of patients and their needs. New drugs, with new dosage profiles and mechanisms of action, constantly enter the market, requiring nurses to continually update their skills. At the same time, patients present an increasingly wide range of conditions, clinical histories, and responses to treatments, necessitating ever greater attention and personalization in medication administration. We cannot forget the context in which nurses operate. The pressures of a high-intensity hospital environment, with its multiple distractions and urgencies, make precision even more crucial. Technology, although it can offer tools to reduce errors, does not eliminate the need for human judgment, intuition, and competence. The machine may suggest a dosage, but it is the nurse who must evaluate its appropriateness in relation to the overall clinical picture of the patient. Finally, dosage calculation is not a solitary activity. It relies on a network of collaboration among healthcare professionals, including physicians, pharmacists, and other specialists. Effective communication, knowledge sharing, and continuous education are essential pillars to ensure that each administered dose is not only mathematically correct but also clinically appropriate and in service of the patient's overall well-being. In summary, dosage calculation is a manifestation of the nurse's deep commitment to safety, care, and professional integrity. Every dose administered represents a promise: the promise to provide evidence-based, personalized, ethical, and high-quality care. And in this commitment, nurses assert themselves not only as competent technicians but as essential custodians of human well-being in the healthcare landscape.

# 2. Fundamentals of Mathematics

**Fundamentals of Mathematics** At the core of any dosage calculation in nursing lies a solid understanding of fundamental mathematical principles. These concepts are crucial not only for performing calculations correctly but also for understanding the "why" behind each calculation, thereby providing safe and effective patient care.

**Basic Mathematical Operations** The four primary mathematical operations - addition, subtraction, multiplication, and division - form the foundation of any calculation. Here's a brief overview:

- **Addition:** This is the process of adding two or more numbers. In the context of medications, it can be useful when calculating the total dose of a medication to be administered during a specific period.

- **Subtraction:** This operation involves subtracting one number from another. It is essential when calculating differences, such as the remaining dose of a medication after a certain administration.

- **Multiplication:** This is the process of increasing one number by another specified number. This operation is common when calculating doses based on a patient's weight.

- **Division:** This operation divides one number by another. It is used, for example, when determining the dose per unit of a medication. These operations are the basis of mathematics, and every healthcare professional must master them to ensure accuracy in medication administration.
**Fractions, Percentages, Decimals** In addition to basic operations, having a clear understanding of fractions, percentages, and decimals is fundamental for dosage calculation.
- **Fraction:** A fraction represents a part of a whole. For example, if a medication needs to be administered as "1/2" of a tablet, that "1/2" is a fraction. Fractions can be converted to decimals and vice versa, and the ability to do this smoothly is crucial in dosage calculation.
- **Percentages:** A percentage is another way to represent a part of a whole, but on a scale of 100. Saline solutions, for example, might be available in various concentration percentages, such as 0.9%. Understanding how to convert percentages to fractions and decimals can be essential, especially when working with different concentrations.
- **Decimals:** A decimal is a number that represents a part of a whole using a decimal point. Many dosage calculations will result in decimal numbers, and nurses must be sure to

interpret the decimal point position correctly to ensure dose accuracy.

Mastering these mathematical concepts is key to performing dosage calculations safely and effectively. Errors can have serious consequences, making this mastery not just useful but vital in the clinical context. Mathematics, although it may seem like an abstract and sometimes intimidating subject for many, proves to be a lifeline in everyday nursing practice. Every operation, from the simplest dosage of a liquid medication to the calculation of a complex infusion regimen, depends on the nurse's ability to accurately apply fundamental mathematical principles.

Basic mathematical operations, however rudimentary they may seem, form the basis of every more advanced calculation. Addition, for instance, might be used when summing the total amount of medication administered in a 12-hour shift, while subtraction may come into play when subtracting an already administered dose from a prescribed total dose.

Multiplication becomes critical, especially when calculating doses based on specific patient parameters. Imagine, for instance, a medication that needs to be dosed based on the patient's weight. Multiplying the specific dosage (expressed perhaps in mg per kg) by the patient's actual weight becomes essential.

Similarly, division is fundamental when working with different units of measurement or when a total dose needs to be divided into multiple administrations. A medication prescribed to be administered in three equal doses throughout the day would require division of the total dosage by three.

Fractions, percentages, and decimals, while concepts many people remember from school, take on an entirely new and vital meaning in nursing practice. A medication might be prescribed in a fraction of a standard dose, such as 1/4 or 3/4 of a tablet. Or you might encounter it in solutions with specific percentages, such as a 5% solution.

Understanding the relationship between fractions, percentages, and decimals is essential. Quickly converting between these forms can make the difference between a correct dose and a potential overdose. For example, knowing that a 10% solution is equivalent to a 0.10 or 1/10 solution can be vital when preparing a medication or diluting a drug.

In the real world, nurses may also deal with technological tools like infusion pumps that require input in specific formats. Some pumps might require dosages in milliliters per hour, while others might require dosages in micrograms per minute. Understanding how to convert between these units and how to use decimals in the process is crucial to ensure that the patient receives the correct amount of medication.

Furthermore, it's not just about understanding the numbers, but also comprehending the context in which they are applied. A nurse must know not only "how" to perform the calculation but also "why" they are doing it. This deep understanding of the context and the rationale behind each calculation ensures that patient care always remains at the core of nursing practice.

As technology continues to advance and tools become more sophisticated, mathematics remains a fundamental cornerstone. Regardless of how advanced the tools become, the nurse's understanding and correct application of mathematical principles will always be crucial. And in a field where precision can mean the difference between life and death, mathematics in all its forms plays an irreplaceable role in ensuring patient safety and care.

Mathematics in nursing practice goes far beyond mere calculations; it's also a matter of interpretation and understanding nuances. Clinical practice often places nurses in situations where a calculation is not just a formula to solve but a set of clinical circumstances to consider.

Consider, for example, patient variability. A dosage that works for one patient may not work for another. Factors like age, metabolism, renal or hepatic function, and other comorbidities can influence the pharmacokinetics and pharmacodynamics of drugs. This means that even if two patients receive the same weight-based dosage, the actual amount of the drug reaching the site of action and its effectiveness can vary significantly.

Fractions, percentages, and decimals play a significant role in this context. For example, it might be necessary to adjust a dosage based on compromised renal function. If a patient, for instance, has only 50% of normal renal function, this may translate into a need to reduce the dosage of a drug eliminated by the kidneys by a corresponding percentage.

Pharmacogenomics also comes into play. As this field of medicine develops, we are discovering that individual genetic variations can influence a patient's response to certain drugs. In some cases, these genetic variations can be quantified in terms of percentages, and nurses may need to apply this knowledge in practice, adjusting doses or administration timings based on specific genetic profiles.

In addition to drug dosages, nurses also find themselves having to calculate other aspects of care, such as a patient's fluid balance. Monitoring fluid intake and output, translating these values into percentage variations, and interpreting what these variations mean for the patient are all skills that require a solid mathematical foundation.

Another crucial aspect is dilution. Many drugs are supplied in a concentrated form that needs to be diluted before use. Understanding how to convert concentrations, such as moving from a 10% solution to a 5% solution, requires an understanding not only of basic mathematical operations but also the laws of concentration and dilution.

And what makes all of this even more challenging is the need to perform these calculations often in high-pressure situations where time is of the essence. The ability to perform calculations quickly and accurately while considering the patient's overall clinical picture cannot be underestimated.

As new drugs and therapies develop, and medicine becomes increasingly personalized, the need for nurses to have a solid mathematical foundation and apply these concepts in practice becomes ever more imperative. Mathematics, in the context of patient care, serves as a bridge between the science and art of nursing practice, enabling nurses to provide optimal care based on sound principles and concrete evidence.

In the context of nursing, mathematical fundamentals are not simply numbers or abstract formulas, but tangible tools that guide crucial clinical decisions every day. These basic mathematical operations - addition, subtraction, multiplication, division - as well as the understanding and manipulation of fractions, percentages, and decimals, are the cornerstones that underpin safe and effective nursing practice. Every single calculation has direct implications for the health and well-being of the patient. A miscalculated dose or misinterpreted percentage can lead to serious consequences, from unwanted side effects to potentially life-threatening situations. This is why mathematics, in its apparent simplicity, becomes a responsibility of vital importance. Every nurse, regardless of their field of specialization or the context in which they work, relies on these fundamental concepts to ensure the correct administration of medications, accurately monitor fluid balance, customize therapies based on specific patient needs, and much more.

Furthermore, beyond the mere execution of calculations, the critical skill of the nurse also lies in the ability to interpret and apply these numbers in a clinical context. This means having a holistic view of the patient, considering all aspects - from physiological status to comorbidities, from genetic variations to personal preferences - and integrating this information with a solid mathematical foundation.

In conclusion, mathematical fundamentals are not just a technical competence but a central aspect of the art and science of nursing. They represent a balance between the precision of numbers and the humanity of care, ensuring that every clinical decision is informed, accurate, and, above all, patient-centered. In an era of advanced and personalized medicine, mathematics remains one of the most powerful tools available to nurses to ensure high-quality care and save human lives.

### 3. Measurement Systems • Metric, Imperial, Apothecary: Conversions and Differences.

Measurement systems play a fundamental role in the healthcare field, especially in drug dosage calculations and therapy administration. Nurses must have a clear understanding of these systems and their interrelationships to ensure patient safety.

**Metric:** The metric system is one of the most universally adopted measurement systems, especially in the scientific and medical fields. It is based on units of measure such as the meter, gram, and liter and uses multiples and submultiples of ten, such as the kilogram (1000 grams) or milliliter (0.001 liters). It is an intuitive and easily scalable system, making it ideal for many medical applications. For example, most liquid medications are prescribed in milligrams (mg) or milliliters (ml).

**Imperial:** The imperial system, often referred to as the standard system, has its roots in traditional units of measurement used in the past in Great Britain and the United States. Some of the most common units include the pound, ounce, pint, and gallon. Although this system is less common in the medical field compared to the metric system, nurses in the United States may still need to use or convert it, especially when interpreting old prescriptions or working with patients who are more familiar with these units.

**Apothecary:** This is one of the oldest measurement systems and has its origins in European traditions of pharmaceutical preparation. Although it is largely obsolete in many parts of the world, some of its units are still used in specific contexts. Common units in the apothecary system include the grain, dram, and minim. Its complexity lies in non-standardized conversions between various units, which can vary depending on the substance being measured.

Conversions between these systems are crucial. For example, knowing how to convert milligrams to grains or ounces to milliliters can be essential in situations where different measurement systems are used. There are conversion tables and tools that nurses can use, but having a basic familiarity with the most common conversions can expedite the process and reduce the risk of errors.

The differences between these systems go beyond simple units of measure. Each system has its own history, culture, and logic. While the metric system is based on decimals and lends itself well to use in scientific contexts due to its uniformity, the imperial and apothecary systems have roots in historical traditions and practices that can make conversions less intuitive.

In summary, understanding measurement systems and their interrelationships is a fundamental element of nursing practice. Each system has its peculiarities, and as the world moves increasingly toward adopting the metric system, the ability to navigate and convert between these systems remains a valuable skill to ensure patient safety.

Choosing the right measurement system can directly impact the effectiveness and safety of pharmacological therapies. While some medications are produced and distributed according to a specific measurement system, others may require conversions depending on the country of production or healthcare institution. In modern times, the globalization of pharmaceutical production and distribution can lead to situations where a doctor in one country may prescribe a medication based on one system, while the nurse may have access to a drug that uses a different measurement system. These discrepancies can introduce margins of error that can have serious consequences for patients.

Moreover, it's not just about medications. The tools used in daily practice, such as syringes, infusion pumps, and diagnostic equipment, may have scales based on various measurement systems. A syringe measuring in milliliters may not have the same graduations as a syringe measuring in ounces, even though both are used for liquid administration.

Another aspect to consider is the training and education of healthcare professionals. Not all nurses and doctors are trained in the same measurement systems. For example, a nurse trained in Europe may be much more familiar with the metric system, while one trained in the United States may have a deeper knowledge of the imperial system. These differences in education can lead to communication challenges, especially in international or multicultural contexts.

## Historical and Cultural Considerations

There are also historical and cultural considerations. While the apothecary system may be considered obsolete in many modern contexts, it has had a significant impact on medical practice for centuries. Understanding the origins and reasons behind specific units of measurement can help healthcare professionals better comprehend their application and significance.

Terminology can also vary. For example, what is known as a "gallon" in the United States has a different volume than a "gallon" in the United Kingdom, despite sharing the same name. These subtle differences can cause confusion if not correctly identified and addressed.

Furthermore, the ongoing evolution of medical technology can lead to changes in the measurement systems used. With the advent of digitization and automation, there may be a growing standardization toward the metric system. However, this does not eliminate the need for healthcare professionals to be versatile and have a deep knowledge of all systems.

In the field of nursing, this depth of understanding is crucial to avoid dosage errors, which can have harmful or potentially fatal side effects. In this context, the ability to convert quickly and accurately between systems, along with the ability to recognize when a conversion is necessary, becomes an invaluable skill.

In the complex web of healthcare, the interactions between healthcare professionals, patients, and medications are inherently linked to measurement systems. This complexity is amplified by the diverse geographical origins of patients, different drug manufacturers, and various practices adopted in healthcare facilities worldwide.

In some cases, a patient may have prescriptions from different countries due to travel or dual residency. These prescriptions may use different measurement systems, requiring nurses to perform multiple and accurate conversions to ensure patient safety. These challenges can be further complicated if the patient is unable to communicate clearly due to language or cultural barriers.

Beyond prescriptions, even the equipment used in patient care can vary based on the measurement system. For example, a blood pressure monitor may use millimeters of mercury (mmHg) as a unit of measurement in one region, while another may use a different unit in another region. These differences can influence result interpretation and subsequent diagnosis or treatment.

Moreover, globalization has led to increased mobility of healthcare professionals. A nurse trained in Asia may find themselves working in Europe or North America. This diversity in education may lead to differences in how healthcare professionals approach and interpret measurement systems, especially in emergency situations where speed and accuracy are essential.

Continuous education and professional development become essential. With the advent of new drugs, techniques, and equipment, nurses must constantly refresh their skills and expand their knowledge of measurement systems. Workshops, seminars, and online courses can provide nurses with the resources needed to stay up-to-date with the latest trends and best practices.

Technology can also offer solutions. Conversion applications and software are increasingly available and can assist nurses in making conversions quickly and accurately. However, these tools do not replace the need for a solid fundamental understanding. In fact, excessive reliance on technology can lead to complacency and potential errors if the tools are unavailable or malfunction.

Patient culture and expectations are another factor to consider. While a patient may be accustomed to receiving medication doses in a certain unit of measure in their home country, they may become confused or concerned if a nurse in another country uses a different system. Effective communication and patient education become crucial in ensuring the patient's understanding and trust in the care process.

At its core, nursing practice is centered on patient care and safety. In the intricate web of modern healthcare, understanding and navigating measurement systems become an integral part of this mission. While it may seem like a technical detail, its importance in ensuring effective and safe care cannot be underestimated. The theme of measurement systems in healthcare is not merely a technical or bureaucratic matter but represents a fundamental pillar in terms of safety and the effectiveness of care. Mastery of different systems - metric, imperial, and apothecary - and the ability to move agilely between them are essential skills for every healthcare professional, especially for nurses who are at the forefront of drug administration and patient monitoring.

In this regard, globalization and the mobility of patients and healthcare professionals have made this issue even more relevant. We live in an era where a patient can be diagnosed in one country, receive treatment in another, and then be monitored at home in a completely different nation. This geographic and clinical complexity implies that measurement systems cannot be viewed in isolation from each other. The ability to convert, interpret, and apply units of measurement appropriately in different situations is essential to ensure accurate and personalized care.

The aspect of communication should also not be overlooked. Transparency and clarity in communication between professionals and patients are crucial to prevent errors and misunderstandings. When a patient does not understand medication doses or has uncertainties about the measurement systems used, there is a tangible risk of non-adherence to therapies or improper administration. This underscores the importance of effective training and ongoing education for healthcare professionals, not only in clinical techniques but also in the ability to communicate this information in an understandable manner to patients.

In conclusion, while technology and digital tools can provide support in this area, they cannot replace the deep knowledge and critical understanding by nurses. These professionals must be armed not only with the skills to perform conversions and calculations but also with the wisdom to recognize when and how to use each system, always keeping the ultimate goal in mind: providing safe, effective, and compassionate care. Mastery of measurement systems, therefore, is not just a matter of numbers but represents an ethical and professional commitment in the interest of patient well-being.

## 4. Principles of Pharmacology • Introduction to Pharmacology and Terminology

Pharmacology, as a field of study, delves deeply into the interaction between drugs and living organisms. It explores how chemical substances, both natural and synthetic, influence physiological and biochemical processes. This branch of medicine is fundamental for understanding pharmacotherapy, especially for ensuring that drugs are administered safely and effectively.

### Introduction to Pharmacology

At the core of pharmacology, there are key concepts concerning how drugs are absorbed, distributed, metabolized, and eliminated from the body – often summarized with the acronym ADME. These processes are crucial to understand how and when a drug will exert its effect and how long it will remain active in the body.

In addition to these fundamental processes, pharmacology examines the reactions that drugs have with specific receptors present in cells. These reactions can be described in terms of affinity (how strong the bond is between the drug and the receptor) and efficacy (how well the drug activates or inhibits the receptor). Understanding these interactions is essential for developing new drugs and predicting how they will react in the human body.

**Basic Terminology in Pharmacology**
• **Drug:** A chemical substance used to diagnose, treat, or prevent diseases or disorders, or to relieve their symptoms.
• **Pharmacodynamics:** Studies the effect of drugs on the body, i.e., how drugs exert their therapeutic effects and which mechanisms are involved.
• **Pharmacokinetics:** Analyzes the movement of drugs within the body, including absorption, distribution, metabolism, and elimination.
• **Agonist:** A drug that activates a receptor and produces a response.
• **Antagonist:** A drug that binds to a receptor but does not activate it, thus preventing its activation by an agonist.
• **Biodisponibility:** The percentage of a administered drug that reaches systemic

circulation in an unchanged form and can therefore exert a therapeutic effect. • **Half-life:** The time required to reduce a drug's concentration in the bloodstream by 50%. Understanding these terms and concepts is essential for those working in the healthcare field, particularly for nurses, as it allows them to comprehend the science behind drug administration and provide safe and effective care to patients. Pharmacology is not just the study of drugs per se but represents the synergy between science, medicine, and patient care. Every nurse must have a strong foundation in pharmacology to make informed decisions and provide optimal care.

Pharmacology, being a vast and complex field, is continuously evolving with the discovery of new drugs and a deeper understanding of the molecular and cellular mechanisms that regulate the body's response to these substances.

At the heart of pharmacology lies the concept of selectivity. While in theory, a drug should act only on a specific target to produce a desired effect, in practice, many drugs have effects on more than one type of receptor or channel. This can lead to side effects. For example, a drug designed to lower blood pressure by acting on a specific type of receptor in the heart might also influence other receptors in the body, leading to undesired effects such as dry mouth or fatigue. Routes of drug administration are another fundamental aspect. Each route, whether oral, intramuscular, intravenous, topical, has its peculiarities in terms of onset of action, bioavailability, and potential complications. Nurses must be particularly aware of these differences. For instance, a drug administered intravenously has an almost immediate action and 100% bioavailability but also carries a higher risk of rapid adverse reactions.

An intriguing and rapidly evolving area of pharmacology concerns biologic drugs and gene therapy. Biologic drugs are manufactured using living organisms and often target very specific sites in the body. Unlike traditional drugs, which are often small chemical molecules, biologic drugs can be proteins or nucleic acids. This specificity can reduce side effects but can also pose challenges in terms of production, storage, and administration.

Gene therapy, on the other hand, aims to treat diseases by introducing, removing, or modifying the genetic material inside an individual's cells. While the potential of these therapies is immense, there are still numerous technical and ethical challenges to overcome.

Another critical area is pharmacogenetics, which explores how individual genetic variations can influence a person's response to drugs. This can have profound implications for personalizing pharmacological therapy. For example, a patient may have a genetic variant that makes them more susceptible to the side effects of a particular drug, or that increases or decreases the drug's effectiveness. Pharmacogenetics seeks to identify these variants to allow physicians to prescribe the most suitable and safe drug for each patient.

**Finally, we cannot overlook the importance of ethics in pharmacology. With the increasing ability to create powerful and targeted drugs, questions arise about who should have access to these drugs, how they should be tested, and whether there are ethical limits to what pharmacology can or should seek to achieve.**

Within the vast landscape of pharmacology, it's also interesting to examine the environmental impact of drugs. When we think of drugs, we often focus on their direct effects on individuals, overlooking the fact that once excreted or eliminated, these compounds can enter the environment. This can occur through the sewer system, where incompletely metabolized drugs can end up in water bodies and affect aquatic fauna. There are studies showing how certain fish species can be influenced by the presence of drugs such as hormones or antidepressants in water bodies.

Another critical topic relates to drug resistance. Antibiotics, for example, have been a cornerstone of modern medicine, but their overuse or inappropriate use has led to the emergence of antibiotic-resistant bacterial strains. This antibiotic resistance represents one of the major challenges to global health, with previously treatable conditions becoming life-threatening again.

In the context of globalization, it's also essential to consider drug access. While industrialized nations have broad access to a wide range of drugs, many regions of the world, especially developing countries, face significant challenges. These include limited availability of essential treatments, prohibitive costs, and the presence of counterfeit or low-quality drugs. The issue of equitable drug access is an ethical challenge that requires attention at both the national and international levels.

Another area of interest concerns so-called "orphan drugs," which are drugs intended to treat rare diseases. Due to the limited number of patients with these conditions, it's not always economically advantageous for pharmaceutical companies to invest in research and development for these treatments. However, for patients with these diseases, such drugs can represent their only hope for treatment. As a society, how do we balance economic needs with the ethical necessity of providing care to all?

An area gaining increasing attention is the interaction between drugs and the human microbiome, the vast community of microorganisms living within our bodies. It's believed that the microbiome influences drug response, metabolism, and even susceptibility to side effects. This suggests that in the future, we may need to consider not only a patient's genetic profile but also the composition of their microbiome when prescribing drugs.

Drug-drug interactions present another challenge. While a single drug might have a well-defined safety profile when used alone, its combined use with other drugs could produce unexpected or enhanced effects. With the increasing prevalence of polypharmacy, especially in elderly populations, the ability to predict and manage these interactions becomes essential.

Patient education about pharmacotherapy is an area that deserves special attention. Often, a patient's understanding of the use, side effects, and potential benefits of a drug can directly influence their adherence to treatment. Studies have shown that patients who understand why they are taking a particular drug and the potential benefits derived from it are more likely to adhere to the therapeutic regimen. This awareness underscores the importance for nurses and other healthcare providers to provide clear and understandable drug education.

Technology is playing an increasingly prominent role in modern pharmacology. Digital applications, for instance, can help patients monitor their drug intake, recognize side effects, and report any anomalies to their healthcare providers. These apps can also provide reminders for drug intake, ensuring that patients don't skip doses and maintain a consistent therapeutic regimen.

An intriguing perspective also involves the use of artificial intelligence (AI) in drug discovery and development. The computational power of modern AI technologies allows for the analysis of extensive datasets to identify potential pharmaceutical compounds and predict their efficacy and safety in biological models. This could revolutionize the speed and efficiency with which new drugs are brought to the market.

**The ethics of clinical experimentation is another central issue in pharmacology. To determine the efficacy and safety of a new drug, it is necessary to test it on human subjects. This raises ethical questions concerning informed consent, participant selection, and potential risks and benefits. Furthermore, with the increasing globalization of clinical research, issues emerge regarding drug testing in countries with different ethical standards or limited resources.**

Another aspect to consider is the evolution of diseases themselves. As society changes, so do diseases. For example, with the global rise in obesity, there is expected to be an increased need for drugs to treat related complications, such as diabetes and cardiovascular diseases. Similarly, an aging population may lead to a greater demand for drugs to address age-related conditions like Alzheimer's or osteoporosis. Finally, the role of culture and societal perceptions of drugs cannot be overlooked. The use of drugs can be viewed very differently in various cultures. In some contexts, there may be greater trust in traditional medicines compared to modern drugs, while in others, there may be a tendency to overuse or misuse certain medications. Understanding these cultural dynamics can be essential for the effective administration and prescription of drugs in an increasingly globalized society.

In conclusion, pharmacology is not just the study of substances that influence biological processes but represents a nexus of science, society, ethics, and culture. Every drug carries a story, from the initial idea to discovery, clinical testing, and finally its introduction into the pharmaceutical market. This journey is not solely driven by the pursuit of therapeutic efficacy but also by economic, ethical, and social considerations. Pharmacological terminology, as the first point of introduction for anyone delving into this discipline, is crucial not only for understanding the "how" and "why" behind a drug's action but also for effective communication within the medical community and with patients. This terminology reflects the complexity and depth of the field, encompassing everything from metabolic pathways to drug-drug interactions, side effects, and adverse reactions.

However, beyond technical terminology, it is essential to understand the broader contexts in which pharmacology operates. This includes the importance of patient education, the evolution of diseases, societal perceptions of drugs, and the impact of globalization. Pharmacology is not an isolated science; it is deeply intertwined with the fabric of society and influenced by cultural, economic, and technological changes.

In an era where information is increasingly accessible but often distorted or misleading, the ability to communicate clear and accurate information about pharmacology is more critical than ever. And as we strive to develop new drugs to address emerging diseases and global health challenges, we must also critically reflect on the broader implications of our choices and actions. In summary, pharmacology, with its terminology and principles, is a lens through which we can see not only the microscopic world of cellular processes but also the macroscopic dynamics of global society and the ethical challenges we face.


## 5. Prescription Reading: How to Interpret Medical Prescriptions

Interpreting a medical prescription correctly is crucial to ensure patient safety and treatment effectiveness. Prescriptions can appear complex due to the use of abbreviations, medical terminology, and specific notations. However, understanding prescriptions is essential for nurses, pharmacists, and other healthcare professionals, as well as for the patients themselves.

**Origins and History of Prescriptions**

Prescriptions have a long history dating back to ancient civilizations when they were inscribed on clay tablets or written on papyrus. Over time, the structure and format of prescriptions became more standardized, especially with the advent of modern medical practice. Although prescriptions are often generated electronically today, traditional terminology and abbreviations are still widely used.

**Key Elements of Prescriptions**

Prescriptions usually include:

- **Patient Name and Identifying Details:** Ensures that the medicine is provided to the right person.
- **Date:** Indicates when the prescription was written. Some prescriptions have an expiration date after which they can no longer be dispensed.
- **Drug Name:** This can be the generic name or the brand name.
- **Dosage:** Specifies the quantity of the drug the patient should take.
- **Route of Administration:** For example, oral, intramuscular, topical.
- **Frequency:** Specifies how often the patient should take the drug, such as twice a day, daily, etc.
- **Duration:** For how long the patient should take the medication.

- **Specific Instructions:** For example, "take with food" or "avoid sun exposure."
- **Doctor's Signature and Contact Details:** Important for verification and any questions.

**Common Abbreviations in Prescriptions**

Understanding abbreviations is essential for correctly interpreting a prescription. For example:

- **q.d.:** every day
- **b.i.d.:** twice a day
- **t.i.d.:** three times a day
- **q.i.d.:** four times a day
- **p.r.n.:** as needed
- **a.c.:** before meals
- **p.c.:** after meals

**Challenges in Prescription Interpretation**

Despite efforts to make prescriptions clear and understandable, issues can arise. For example, illegible handwriting or improper use of abbreviations can lead to medication dispensing errors. With the increase in electronic prescriptions, many of these problems are decreasing, but challenges can still emerge, such as system errors or compatibility issues between different software.

**Patients' Role in Prescription Interpretation**

While healthcare professionals play a key role in interpreting and implementing prescriptions, patients also have a responsibility. It's important for patients to understand their prescription, seek clarification when they have doubts, and carefully follow instructions. Moreover, they should always check medication labels when receiving medicine to ensure it matches what was prescribed.

In summary, interpreting a prescription correctly is an essential skill to ensure that medications are administered safely and effectively. It requires a combination of understanding medical terminology, attention to detail, and clear communication among physicians, pharmacists, nurses, and patients.

**Interpreting medical prescriptions is an ongoing challenge, not only due to the intrinsic complexity of the information contained but also because of the potentially dangerous consequences of misinterpretation.**

## Technological Trends and Electronic Prescriptions

Technological trends have introduced electronic prescriptions, aiming to reduce human errors. However, these systems are not without challenges. Software interfaces must be intuitive and minimize the possibility of entering incorrect data. Although the legibility of handwriting is no longer an issue, electronic prescriptions may pose integration problems between different hospital or pharmacy systems, creating barriers in information transmission.

## Importance of Continuous Education

Given the constant evolution of pharmacological therapies and clinical recommendations, it is essential for healthcare professionals to engage in continuous education. This helps ensure not only an understanding of new available therapies but also familiarity with new or less common terms and abbreviations that may appear in prescriptions.

## Communication Among Healthcare Professionals

It is crucial that there is open and clear communication among various healthcare professionals. For example, if a pharmacist has doubts about a prescription, they should feel free to contact the prescribing physician for clarification. This type of interprofessional communication can prevent potentially dangerous errors and ensure patient safety.

## Patients' Role and Functional Illiteracy

While healthcare professionals have the primary responsibility to ensure the clarity of prescriptions, patients also play a crucial role. It is estimated that a significant percentage of the population suffers from "functional illiteracy," which means they may not fully comprehend written instructions. This emphasizes the need to ensure that prescriptions are written clearly and understandably, and that patients receive adequate education on how to read and interpret instructions.

## Prescriptions in Different Languages

In an increasingly globalized world, it's not uncommon for patients to receive care in a country where they do not speak the native language. This poses the challenge of ensuring that prescriptions are understandable even for those who do not speak the language in which they are written. Some hospitals and clinics are implementing automatic translation systems or using human translators to ensure prescription clarity for all patients, regardless of their native language.

## Compliance with Regulations and Privacy

With the advent of electronic prescriptions, concerns about data privacy and security also arise. It is essential for such systems to comply with privacy regulations and ensure the security of patients' sensitive information.

In conclusion, while interpreting prescriptions may seem like a straightforward translation of information from one document to another, it is, in fact, a complex interplay of skills, communication, and technology. Every aspect of this process has profound implications for patient safety and well-being.

## Management of Medication Prescriptions: A Complex Arena

Cultural Safety and Error Reduction

Prescription-related errors are a major concern in the healthcare sector. To reduce such errors, many healthcare facilities are adopting a culture of safety, emphasizing the importance of openly discussing errors, analyzing them, and implementing corrective measures. This type of culture encourages healthcare providers to report errors without fear of repercussions, enabling a more effective response.

## Role of Technology and Artificial Intelligence

With the evolution of technology, artificial intelligence (AI) is playing an increasing role in prescription management. There are systems that use AI to detect potential drug interactions, incorrect dosages, or other anomalies in a prescription before it reaches the patient. These systems can act as an additional layer of verification, reducing the risk of human errors.

## Interpersonal Dynamics and Patient-Centered Care

The importance of effective communication between the physician and the patient cannot be emphasized enough. The physician must ensure that the patient understands not only the dosage and frequency of medication but also the reason for the prescription, potential side effects, and potential interactions with other drugs. This requires time, empathy, and attention.

## Access to Care Issues and Medication Costs

Prescriptions, while a fundamental part of a patient's care plan, can pose problems if patients cannot afford the prescribed medications. In many nations, the high cost of drugs presents a significant barrier for many patients. Healthcare providers must be aware of these challenges and seek, where possible, more cost-effective alternatives or assistance programs that can help patients obtain the medications they need.

## Cultural Awareness and Sensitivity

In an increasingly diverse society, healthcare providers must also be aware of cultural differences that can influence the perception and use of medications. For example, some cultures may have traditional beliefs or practices that influence their willingness to take certain drugs.

Understanding and respecting these differences is essential for providing effective care.

## The Need for Ongoing Education

As in many sectors of the medical field, the realm of prescriptions is continually evolving. New drugs are developed, guidelines change, and technologies advance. To keep pace with these innovations, healthcare providers must engage in continuous education, participating in seminars, courses, and other educational opportunities.

## The Same Prescription in Different Contexts

An often overlooked aspect of prescriptions is how they can vary depending on the context. For example, a prescription in a hospital setting may differ slightly from one in an outpatient clinic or a nursing home. Nurses and other professionals must be attentive to these nuances and adapt their practices accordingly.

In conclusion, prescription management goes beyond merely reading and interpreting a document. It involves a deep understanding of medicine, technology, communication, and interpersonal dynamics, all interwoven in a delicate balance with the primary goal of patient safety and well-being.

## Reading and Interpreting Medical Prescriptions

Reading and interpreting medical prescriptions are fundamental activities in nursing practice and healthcare in general. Properly interpreting prescriptions ensures that patients receive the appropriate therapies, minimizing the risk of medical errors and associated complications. However, as we've explored, this practice is not simple and requires multidisciplinary skills.

Key elements in interpreting prescriptions:

1. **Accuracy:** The importance of reading and interpreting every detail of a prescription, from drug identification to dosage and administration frequency, cannot be emphasized enough. Each element must be examined with the utmost care.

2. **Effective Communication:** Collaboration among various healthcare professionals, including physicians, nurses, pharmacists, and therapists, is crucial. Each professional has a specific role in the process, and their collaboration ensures that the patient receives the most appropriate therapy.

3. **Patient Education:** It is not enough to simply give the patient the prescribed medicine. It is essential to inform the patient about why that particular drug was prescribed, its potential side effects, and how and when to take it. This

ensures that the patient is an active partner in their care.

4. **Use of Technology:** While technology has simplified many aspects of the process, it has also introduced new challenges. Healthcare providers must be adequately trained to use electronic prescription systems and other digital tools, ensuring patient data security and privacy.

5. **Cultural Awareness:** We live in a globalized world with an increasing diversity of patients from various cultural backgrounds. The ability to understand and respect diverse cultural perspectives and beliefs regarding medicine and healthcare is essential.

6. **Continuous Improvement:** Medicine is an evolving field, with new drugs, treatments, and guidelines emerging regularly. Healthcare providers must engage in continuous learning and updates to ensure they deliver the most current and evidence-based care to their patients. In conclusion, interpreting medical prescriptions is a complex task that plays a crucial role in patient care. It requires precision, communication, education, and a deep understanding of both medicine and the individuals it is intended for. Its proper execution ensures not only the health and safety of patients but also strengthens the trust between patients

and healthcare providers, a key element for successful care.

# 6. Oral Dose Calculations: Liquids, Tablets, Capsules

*Oral Dose Calculations: Liquids, Tablets, Capsules*
When we talk about oral dose calculations, we refer to the process of determining the exact amount of medication to administer to a patient via the oral route. This is a crucial skill for nurses and other healthcare professionals as it ensures that patients receive the correct dose of medication, thus avoiding overdosing or underdosing that could have serious health consequences.

**Liquids** Medications in liquid form are often prescribed in milliliters (ml) or other liquid measurement units. The drug's concentration in the liquid is generally expressed as an amount of drug per unit of volume, such as mg/ml.

- **Concentration and Volume:** To determine the correct dose of a liquid medication, nurses must consider both the drug's concentration and the total volume to be administered. For example, if a doctor prescribes 50 mg of a drug, and the available solution has a concentration of

10 mg/ml, the patient should be given 5 ml of that solution.

- **Use of Measuring Tools:** It's essential to use appropriate measuring instruments, such as dosing syringes or graduated cylinders, to ensure accuracy in administration.

**Tablets and Capsules** Tablets and capsules are the most common forms of orally administered drugs and are generally prescribed in milligrams (mg) or other weight measurement units.

- **Dosage:** When administering a drug in tablet or capsule form, it's essential to consider the prescribed dosage and the available dosage for each tablet or capsule. For example, if a dose of 100 mg is prescribed, and 50 mg tablets are available, the patient should take two tablets.

- **Tablet Division:** In some cases, it may be necessary to divide tablets to obtain the correct dose. It's important to use appropriate tools like pill splitters to ensure precise division and avoid incorrect dosages.

- **Capsule Considerations:** Unlike tablets, capsules cannot be divided. If the required dose is not available in a capsule of a certain size, it may be necessary to prescribe a combination of different capsule sizes or consider another form of the drug.

**General Considerations for Oral Dose Calculations:**

- **Standardized Formulas:** Many nurses use standardized formulas to assist in dosage calculations. These formulas take into account the desired dose, the available dose, and the drug's form (liquid, tablet, capsule) to determine the exact quantity to be administered.
- **Verification:** It's essential to always double-check calculations and, if possible, have them reviewed by another healthcare professional. This step reduces the risk of errors.
- **Patient Education:** Once the correct dose is calculated, nurses must instruct patients on how and when to take the medication, as well as potential side effects and interactions with other drugs.

In summary, precise oral dose calculations are a crucial aspect of medication administration. It requires attention to detail, mathematical competence, and a deep understanding of medications and their various forms. When executed correctly, these calculations ensure that patients receive the exact amount of medication needed to treat their conditions, maximizing treatment efficacy and minimizing associated risks.

## Complexities of Oral Dose Calculations

The complexity of oral dose calculations is compounded by several factors that nurses and other healthcare professionals must keep in mind. For example, while medical prescriptions are written with consideration of a patient's weight, age, or other medical conditions, the actual dynamics of drug absorption can vary from individual to individual.

## Bioequivalence and Generic Formulations

Not all tablets or capsules are created equal. Although two drugs may have the same amount of the active ingredient, they could have different release profiles or bioavailability. This is particularly relevant when considering generic drugs compared to their brand-name counterparts. Bioequivalence, meaning that two drugs produce the same effects in the body, is crucial. If a patient switches from a brand-name drug to a generic one or vice versa, close monitoring of the patient's responses and potential dosage adjustments may be necessary.

## Food Interactions

The administration of oral doses can also depend on food. Some medications must be taken on an empty stomach, while others should be taken with food to enhance absorption or reduce side effects. The presence of food can influence the speed and effectiveness of drug absorption. For example, food can delay the absorption of a drug, thus delaying its effects.

## Physiological Variations

Factors such as stomach pH, gastric emptying rate, and the presence of other drugs or substances in the gastrointestinal tract can influence the absorption of an oral drug. Additionally, some individuals may have more permeable intestinal barriers, allowing for faster or increased absorption, while others may have less permeable barriers.

## Tolerance and Adaptation

With continued use, the dose of a drug may need to be adjusted. The body can develop tolerance to certain drugs, meaning that over time, a higher dose may be required to achieve the same effect. This is particularly true for drugs that act on the central nervous system, such as analgesics.

## Controlled-Release Medications

Many drugs today are formulated to be controlled-release or extended-release. This means that the drug is slowly released into the body over several hours, eliminating the need for frequent doses. These formulations can pose challenges in dosage calculations, as dividing or crushing these tablets can alter the release profile, leading to rapid and potentially harmful drug absorption.

Furthermore, splitting tablets is not always straightforward or accurate. Tablets are not always designed to be divided, and even with the use of a pill splitter, they may not split into equal parts. This can result in inconsistent and potentially dangerous dosages.

As technology and research advance, new formulations and administration methods are developed to improve the effectiveness and safety of oral medications. However, this also requires nurses and other healthcare professionals to stay up-to-date and be prepared to adapt to the new challenges these innovations may present.

## Proper Management of Oral Dose Calculations: A Blend of Science and Art

The correct management of oral dose calculations is a symbiosis of science and art. Understanding medications and physiological processes is crucial, but so is the ability to assess each patient as a unique individual with specific needs and reactions.

## Drug Stability and Storage

Medications can degrade or alter if not stored correctly. Light, humidity, temperature, and air can affect a drug's potency and efficacy. For example, some drugs need to be stored in the refrigerator, while others may lose their effectiveness if exposed to direct sunlight. These factors can influence the effective dose a patient receives when taking a drug. Therefore, it's essential for nurses to be aware of each drug's specific storage requirements and to inform patients on how to store their medications correctly at home.

## Genetic Variations and Drug Metabolism

Genetics can play a crucial role in determining how an individual metabolizes a particular drug. Some individuals may have higher or lower enzyme activity, influencing the speed at which a drug is metabolized and eliminated from the body. This may require dosage adjustments to ensure the drug remains in the patient's system for the necessary duration to achieve the desired effect. Pharmacogenomics is an emerging field that explores how individual genetic variations can affect a person's response to drugs.

## Pediatric and Geriatric Dosing

Children and the elderly often require special consideration when it comes to dosage calculations. Children, in particular, have developing organ systems that can affect how they metabolize and respond to medications. On the other hand, the elderly may have reduced kidney or liver function, which can impact drug clearance. These patient groups may also have increased sensitivity to certain side effects.

## Special Formulations

In addition to traditional tablets and capsules, there are numerous other oral formulations, such as suspensions, syrups, lozenges, powders, granules, and so on. Each type has its peculiarities in terms of preparation and administration. For example, a suspension may need to be shaken before use to ensure even distribution of the drug.

## Cultural and Linguistic Knowledge

In today's global society, it's common to encounter patients from various cultures and language backgrounds. Some cultures may have beliefs or practices related to medication intake that differ from traditional Western medicine. Understanding and respecting these differences can help ensure better therapeutic adherence and outcomes for patients.

## Monitoring and Follow-Up

After determining and administering the correct dose, it's crucial to monitor the patient to ensure the drug is having the desired effect and that no side effects occur. This may include regularly measuring drug blood levels, assessing symptoms, or checking with the patient about how they feel. This continuous monitoring may lead to further dosage adjustments or the need to change the medication entirely.

## Multimodal Medications and Polytherapy

In many clinical scenarios, patients are not on a single drug but rather on a combination of medications. Polytherapy, or the concurrent use of multiple drugs, can further complicate oral dosage calculations. Each drug has the potential to interact with another, influencing its effectiveness or increasing the risk of side effects. Some of these interactions can also alter the amount of drug absorbed or the speed at which it is metabolized, necessitating further dosage adjustments.

## Therapeutic Adherence

Even if a dosage is calculated correctly, its effectiveness is pointless if a patient does not adhere to the therapeutic regimen. Non-adherence can occur for various reasons, including side effects, the complexity of the dosage regimen, lack of patient understanding, or economic considerations such as the cost of medications. Nurses often have to act as educators, ensuring that patients understand the importance of their pharmacological regimen and the potential risks of non-adherence.

**Clinical Decision-Making Support Systems**
In the digital age, technology is playing an increasingly significant role in supporting nurses and other healthcare professionals in dosage calculations. Many hospitals and clinics now use electronic decision support systems that can alert nurses to potential dosage errors or drug interactions. However, like any tool, these systems are not infallible and require critical and informed use.

**High-Alert Medications**
Some drugs are particularly high-risk if dosed incorrectly. These "high-alert" medications may include anticoagulants, insulin, opioids, and chemotherapeutics. Due to the potential for severe consequences in the event of a dosage error, these drugs often require additional

checks, such as double-checking by another healthcare professional before administration.

## Awareness of OTC Formulations and Supplements

Not only prescribed medications influence pharmacokinetics and pharmacodynamics, but over-the-counter (OTC) drugs and dietary supplements also do. For example, some supplements, like St. John's Wort, can interact with prescribed medications, altering their effects. Nurses must have a comprehensive understanding of what a patient is taking, not only in terms of prescribed medications but also OTC and supplements.

## Ethical and Legal Implications in Dosage Calculations

Administering medications is not only about science; there are ethical and legal considerations as well. Dosage errors can have serious consequences not only for the patient's health but also for the nurse's career and legal responsibility. Nurses must act with the utmost diligence and care when calculating and administering medications, recognizing the deep trust patients place in them.

## Patient Variability and Treatment Personalization

Every individual is unique in their response to medications. Factors such as age, sex, weight, renal and hepatic function, and comorbidities can all influence an individual's response to a specific dosage. The concept of personalized medicine is gaining recognition as efforts are made to optimize treatment for each patient. This means that nurses, in addition to using standardized formulas for dosage calculations, must also have the ability to adapt these dosages based on the specific needs of the patient.

## Pharmacodynamic Differences

Pharmacodynamics pertains to the effect of the drug on the body. Two patients may metabolize a drug the same way (pharmacokinetics) but may respond differently to the drug due to pharmacodynamic differences. For example, one person may have a greater number of receptors for a particular drug, making them more sensitive to its action. Nurses must be attentive to these varying response levels and be ready to adjust the dosage if necessary.

## Administration Environment

The environment in which a patient receives a drug can also affect its effectiveness. For example, an anxious or stressed patient may metabolize drugs differently than when they are relaxed. The hospital environment itself, with its rhythms and interruptions, can influence the timing and effectiveness of drug administration. Nurses must be attentive not only to the "how" and "how much" of drug administration but also the "where" and "when."

**Ongoing Education and Training**

The field of pharmacology is constantly evolving. New drugs are being developed, old drugs are being withdrawn or replaced, and new research on best dosage practices emerges regularly. To maintain safe and effective practice, nurses must engage in continuous education. This may involve participating in workshops, reading professional journals, or attending training courses sponsored by healthcare institutions.

**Technology and Innovation**

As mentioned earlier, technology plays an ever-increasing role in nursing practice. In addition to decision support systems, there are mobile applications, software, and devices that assist in drug administration and calculation. While these technologies can provide an added level of safety and accuracy, it is essential that nurses do not overly rely on them. Clinical competence and judgment are irreplaceable.

## Feedback and Ongoing Assessment

After the administration of any drug, having a feedback system is vital. This allows monitoring the patient's response, quickly identifying any side effects or adverse reactions, and making any necessary treatment adjustments. This process of continuous assessment ensures that patients receive the best possible care and that any issues are promptly identified and managed.

In summary, oral dosage calculations, while a fundamental skill in nursing practice, are just a small part of a much broader and complex landscape. Drug administration, especially orally, requires a deep understanding of various aspects, from pharmacology to human physiology, from drug interactions to the specific needs of the patient.

Variability among patients introduces a range of challenges. Factors such as age, genetics, comorbidities, and the environment can profoundly influence how an individual responds to a specific drug. Nurses must be prepared not only to calculate the correct dosage but also to anticipate, identify, and manage any atypical responses or side effects.

The importance of ongoing education cannot be emphasized enough. With the continuous development and evolution of drugs, nurses must keep their skills and knowledge up to date. This ensures that patients receive the best possible care and also protects nurses from potential legal and professional liabilities.

Technological innovation provides valuable tools to support nurses, but with this comes the responsibility to use such tools critically and informedly. Overreliance on technology can lead to neglect and errors.

Finally, the importance of a feedback and ongoing assessment system is essential. It's not just about administering the drug but about monitoring and evaluating the effectiveness of treatment, making necessary adjustments based on patient responses and needs.

In conclusion, while the ability to perform accurate oral dosage calculations is crucial, the overall practice of drug administration requires depth of knowledge, critical judgment, and a commitment to continuous learning and adaptation. The health and well-being of patients depend on nurses' ability to competently navigate this complex and dynamic field.

# 7. Parenteral Dose Calculations

**• Injections and Their Dosages**
**Parenteral Dose Calculations: Injections and Their Dosages**
**Types of Injections** Parenteral injections are common methods of drug administration that bypass the gastrointestinal tract. There are several types of injections, each with its own characteristics and techniques:

- **Intradermal (ID):** This type of injection is administered in the dermis, just beneath the epidermis. It is commonly used for allergy tests or the tuberculin test.
- **Subcutaneous (SC or SubQ):** Subcutaneous injections are administered into the fatty tissue just beneath the skin. Common examples include insulin and heparin.
- **Intramuscular (IM):** These injections are administered directly into the muscles. This method allows for the administration of a larger drug dose compared to ID or SubQ techniques. Vaccines and many antibiotics are often administered via this route.
- **Intravenous (IV):** Here, the drug is administered directly into the bloodstream through a vein. This is the quickest method of

drug administration, as it enters the systemic circulation directly.

**Factors to Consider in Parenteral Calculations**

- **Volume:** The amount of solution or drug to be administered. This may be expressed in milliliters (ml) or other units of measurement.
- **Concentration:** Indicates how much active substance is present in a given volume of solution. This is often expressed in mg/ml or similar units.
- **Administration Rate:** For IV injections, the speed at which the drug is administered can be crucial, especially as too rapid an administration can cause side effects.
- **Compatibility:** Before administering two or more drugs together, it's essential to ensure that they are compatible and do not interact adversely.

**Common Formulas** Calculating parenteral dosages can vary depending on the type of drug and the route of administration. However, a common formula is:

*Desired Dose ÷ Available Dose × Available Volume = Volume to Administer*

This calculation helps the nurse determine how much volume of a medicated solution to administer to achieve the desired dose.

**Challenges and Considerations** While dosage calculation is essential, there are other considerations that nurses must keep in mind:

- **Injection Technique:** Each type of injection has a specific technique that must be followed to ensure safe and effective administration.
- **Adverse Reactions:** Reactions can vary depending on the type of drug and route of administration. Nurses must closely monitor patients after administration for any signs of a reaction.
- **Hygiene:** Hygiene is of utmost importance when performing injections to prevent infections and other complications.

Parenteral administration requires precision in both calculation and practice. The nurse's knowledge and competence are essential to ensure that patients receive accurate dosages safely and effectively.

**Site Selection and Injection Placement** The choice of injection site is crucial not only to ensure the drug's effectiveness but also to minimize discomfort and prevent complications.

- **Intradermal (ID):** ID injections are generally administered on the inner forearm, upper arm, or scapula. This is due to the clear visibility of a reaction, such as a raised or reddened area, which can indicate a response to the test.

- **Subcutaneous (SubQ):** Common sites include the abdomen (at least 5 cm away from the navel), the front and outer thigh, the upper outer arm, and the upper back (just below the scapula). Rotation of injection sites is recommended to prevent lipodystrophy.
- **Intramuscular (IM):** IM injections require the drug to penetrate through the skin layer and into the underlying muscle. Common sites for IM injections include the deltoid muscle (arm), vastus lateralis (thigh), and gluteus medius (buttocks). The choice of IM injection site may depend on the quantity of drug to be administered and the patient's age.
- **Intravenous (IV):** The choice of the vein depends on the type and duration of the infusion. Peripheral veins in the forearm are often used for short-term infusions, while more central veins or the use of devices like central catheters may be preferred for long-term or caustic drugs.

**Patient Preparation and Communication**

Patient preparation is a fundamental step before any parenteral administration. Explaining the procedure and the reason for the injection can help reduce patient anxiety. It is also important to assess any previous experiences with injections or adverse reactions.

**Medication Maintenance and Storage**
Proper medication storage is essential to maintain their effectiveness. Many medications, such as insulin, may require refrigeration. Additionally, some medications may have a short shelf life after preparation, making timely administration essential.

**Advanced Techniques and Technology**
The advent of technology has introduced new techniques and equipment for medication administration. For example, infusion pumps can automatically regulate the flow of a drug, ensuring a constant dose. Auto-injector devices provide a safe and consistent way for patients to administer injections to themselves.

The practice of injections and dosage calculations requires in-depth training and a clear understanding of associated responsibilities. While technology can offer tools to facilitate these tasks, the competence, care, and attention of the nurse remain irreplaceable.

**Understanding Pharmacokinetics for Injections**
When administering a drug via a parenteral route, its pharmacokinetics (i.e., how the body absorbs, distributes, metabolizes, and eliminates the drug) can vary significantly from other administration routes. For example, drugs

administered intravenously (IV) enter the bloodstream directly, bypassing the absorption process and providing an immediate effect. This differs from orally administered drugs, which must first pass through the gastrointestinal tract.

**Importance of Sterility**

Sterility is crucial when administering a drug via a parenteral route. Any contamination, whether bacterial, fungal, or viral, can lead to severe complications, including systemic infections. Nurses must ensure that all syringes, needles, and vials are sterile before use. Hand hygiene and the use of sterile gloves are standard procedures to prevent contamination.

**Assessing Patient Response**

After administering a drug via a parenteral route, it is vital to monitor the patient's response. This may include checking vital signs, observing any adverse reactions, and assessing the effectiveness of the treatment. For example, if a patient receives an analgesic, the nurse should periodically assess the patient's pain level.

**Calculating Doses Based on Weight and Age**

For some medications, the dose must be calculated based on the patient's weight or age. For example, children may require proportionally lower doses than adults, but this is not always a simple proportional division. Metabolic variations and differences in drug distribution among tissues can influence the required dose.

## Potential Complications

Even with proper technique, potential complications can arise during parenteral administration. Infiltrations, for instance, occur when an IV drug is inadvertently administered into surrounding tissue instead of the vein. This can cause pain, swelling, and, in some cases, tissue damage. Other potential complications include hematomas, air embolisms, and infections.

## Importance of Documentation

Accurate documentation of each parenteral administration is crucial. This documentation should include the drug's name, dose, route of administration, injection site, time and date of administration, as well as any observed adverse reactions. This information is essential to ensure patient safety and provide a continuous record of care received.

## 8. Calculations for IV Infusions - Drip Rates, Infusion Pumps, and Their Rates

### Fundamentals of IV Infusions

Intravenous (IV) infusion is a common method for administering fluids and medications, providing rapid access to the bloodstream, making it ideal for many treatments.

## Drip Chambers

Drip chambers are components of an IV infusion set that regulate the number of drops per minute (dpm) passing through the infusion line. There are different types of drip chambers:

- **Macro-drip chambers:** Ideal for administering large volumes of fluid, they release larger drops and are generally calibrated for 10, 15, or 20 drops/ml.
- **Micro-drip chambers:** Used for more precise dosages, they release smaller drops, often calibrated for 60 drops/ml.

To calculate the infusion rate, it is essential to know the type of drip chamber used. For example, to infuse 100 ml of a solution in one hour with a drip chamber calibrated at 10 drops/ml, you will have 1000 drops in an hour, approximately 16.7 drops per minute.

## Infusion Pumps

Infusion pumps are electronic devices that regulate the infusion rate of fluids and medications based on a rate set by the operator. These pumps can be programmed to provide a constant or variable flow of drug or fluid.

**Volumetric Pumps**

Volumetric pumps administer a specific quantity of fluid over a predetermined period. They use sensors to monitor and adjust the infusion rate to ensure the correct dose is delivered.

**Syringe Pumps**

Syringe pumps are designed to deliver small volumes of medication at a precise rate using a syringe. They are often used for critical medications such as cardiovascular agents or sedatives.

**Calculation of Infusion Rate**

To determine the IV infusion rate, various calculations are used. Here's a basic example:

If a physician prescribes 500 ml of saline solution to be administered over 4 hours with an infusion set calibrated at 15 drops/ml, the formula would be:

Rate = Volume (ml) / Time (h) × Drip Factor (drops/ml)

Using the provided data:

Rate = 500 ml / 4 h × 15 drops/ml = 1875 drops/h = 31.25 drops/min

So, the solution should be set to infuse at 31.25 drops per minute.

## Factors Affecting Infusion

Several factors can influence the infusion rate, including the viscosity of the liquid, needle size, the patient's blood pressure, and altitude (which can affect atmospheric pressure). Nurses must be aware of these factors and make necessary adjustments to ensure safe and accurate administration.

Proficiency in performing precise calculations for IV infusions is vital for nursing practice. Ensuring that patients receive the right amount of fluid or medication at the correct time can make a difference in terms of patient outcomes and safety.

## Types of IV Infusions

Intravenous infusion is not limited to the administration of fluids alone. There are various types of infusions based on clinical needs:

- **Continuous Infusion:** This involves uninterrupted delivery of fluid or medication. It is commonly used to maintain a stable fluid balance in patients and ensure a constant medication dose.
- **Intermittent Infusion:** This type of infusion is administered at regular intervals. For example, an antibiotic might be given every 6 hours.
- **Bolus Infusion:** This is a rapid method of administration where a significant amount of

medication is injected over a short period. It is used, for example, in emergency situations or when it is necessary to rapidly reach therapeutic drug levels in the patient's bloodstream.

## Components of Infusion Set

Infusion sets consist of various components that aid in facilitating the administration of fluid or medication. These include:

- **Drip Chamber:** This is the transparent section of the infusion set where fluid drops are visible as they fall. It helps nurses calculate the drip rate.
- **Filter:** Many infusion lines contain filters that remove impurities or particles from the fluid before it reaches the patient.
- **Flow Regulator:** This device allows for the adjustment of the infusion rate, ensuring that the patient receives the fluid at the desired pace.
- **Access Port:** Some infusion sets have access ports that allow nurses to administer additional medications without having to insert a new needle or catheter.

## Safety Considerations

While IV infusions are routine, there are several safety considerations that nurses must keep in mind:

- **Drug Incompatibility:** Not all drugs can be mixed together. Nurses must be aware of potential drug interactions and ensure that those administered together are compatible.

- **Infusion Rate:** Administering a drug too quickly can cause side effects in the patient. On the other hand, administering too slowly may not provide the desired therapeutic benefits.
- **Adverse Reactions:** Monitoring patients for any adverse reactions during and after the infusion is essential. This includes allergic reactions, overdosing, and reactions at infusion sites such as redness or swelling.

## Storage and Preparation

It is essential that IV medications and fluids are stored correctly to maintain their effectiveness and safety. For instance, some medications must be stored in a refrigerator and protected from light. Additionally, before infusion, nurses must check the expiration date and ensure that the drug or fluid shows no signs of deterioration, such as cloudiness or separation. Accurate preparation and verification of medications are crucial in preventing medication errors.

## Formulation of IV Medications

While many IV solutions come pre-packaged and ready for use, some require special preparation by the nurse or pharmacist. This preparation may include diluting a concentrated drug or mixing different components to create a customized solution for the patient's needs.

- **Dilution:** Some drugs are provided in concentrated form and need to be diluted before infusion. This process requires precision to ensure the patient receives the correct dose. Inadequate dilution can lead to overdosing or underdosing.

- **Stability:** Once diluted, not all drugs maintain their stability for extended periods. Nurses must be aware of the time during which a drug remains stable after preparation and ensure it is administered within that period.

- **Mixing:** In some situations, it may be necessary to combine multiple drugs or solutions into a single infusion. These combinations must be made following specific protocols to prevent incompatibility and reactions.

## Monitoring the Infusion

IV infusion is not a passive process. It requires continuous vigilance from the nurse to ensure everything proceeds as expected:

- **Site Observation:** Regularly checking the infusion site for signs of inflammation, infection, infiltration, or phlebitis is essential. A change in the color or temperature of the surrounding skin, swelling, or pain are signals of potential issues.

- **Drip Rate Verification:** Even though many infusions are now regulated by electronic pumps, some may still require manual drop counting to ensure the rate is correct.

- **Patient Monitoring:** In addition to the infusion site, nurses must monitor the patient for any signs of adverse reactions, such as changes in heart rate, blood pressure, or respiratory distress.

**Preventing Complications**

As with any medical procedure, there are potential complications associated with IV infusions:

- **Infection:** Since IV infusion introduces substances directly into the bloodstream, there is a risk of infection. Using aseptic techniques during catheter insertion and management can help reduce this risk.

- **Air in the Line:** Accidental introduction of air into the infusion line can potentially cause an air embolism. Although modern IV equipment comes with air bubble detectors, nurses should still be vigilant and ensure the line is free of air before infusion.

- **Infiltration:** Infiltration occurs when IV fluid enters the surrounding tissues instead of the vein. It can cause swelling, pain, and tissue damage.

Ultimately, while technology has made IV infusions safer and more efficient, the nurse's role remains paramount. Through adequate training, evidence-based practice, and continuous vigilance, nurses can ensure their patients receive the best possible care.

## Regulation and Maintenance of IV Equipment

While many IV infusions are controlled by electronic pumps that regulate flow and volume, it is crucial for the nurse to understand how such equipment functions. Different drugs and therapies require specific infusion rates, and correctly setting up the pump is essential to ensure the patient receives therapy as prescribed.

- **Pump Calibration:** Like any electronic device, IV pumps may require periodic calibration to ensure accuracy. This is essential to ensure that the set volume and rate actually correspond to what is delivered to the patient.

- **Power and Backup Batteries:** Power outages or technical failures can compromise the continuous administration of a drug. Having a backup power system is essential, and regularly checking IV pump batteries is crucial.

- **Alarms and Notifications:** Most modern pumps come equipped with alarm systems that alert the nurse to potential issues such as occlusions, air bubbles, or when the IV solution is running low. Nurses should become familiar with these alarms and know how to respond appropriately.

## Infusion Solutions and Components

The type of IV solution and additional components are also key factors in infusions:

- **Solution Types:** There are many different solutions available, including normal saline, lactated Ringer's solution, and dextrose solutions. Each solution has specific indications and contraindications, and nurses must be aware of the differences and appropriate applications.

- **Additives and Medications:** In addition to basic solutions, medications or other additives are often added to the infusion. This may include electrolytes, antibiotics, or other therapeutic agents.

- **Compatibility:** Not all drugs and solutions are compatible with each other. Mixing incompatible agents can lead to precipitates that could clog the catheter or, worse, enter the patient's bloodstream. Nurses should always consult appropriate resources or a pharmacist when mixing drugs or solutions.

**Environment and Patient Positioning**

The context in which the infusion is administered can affect effectiveness and safety:

- **Patient Positioning:** Patient positioning can influence the flow of solution through the catheter. A bent or compressed limb can reduce or block the flow. Nurses should periodically check and reposition the patient as needed.

- **Room Temperature:** In some cases, such as blood transfusions, the solution's temperature may be critical. Solutions that are too cold can cause discomfort or complications for the patient. Therefore, equipment to warm the solution before infusion might be necessary.

- **Hygiene and Cleanliness:** The area around the patient should be kept clean and free from potential contaminants. This is particularly important in areas where infusions are prepared and administered.

All of these aspects emphasize the importance of ongoing training and reflective practice for nurses managing IV infusions. While technology has streamlined many aspects of the process, knowledge and attention to detail remain fundamental to patient safety and effectiveness of IV therapy.

**Monitoring IV Therapy**

Monitoring is a fundamental aspect when administering intravenous therapies. Even though an IV pump may function correctly and the medication can be dosed accurately, the patient's response to the infusion can vary.

- **Vital Sign Monitoring:** Heart rate, blood pressure, oxygen saturation, and respiratory rate are vital indicators of the effect of an infusion. For example, a cardiac stimulant might alter heart rate, while a vasodilator could influence blood pressure.

- **Infusion Site Assessment:** Nurses must regularly inspect the infusion site for signs of inflammation, swelling, redness, or extravasation. The presence of these symptoms may indicate an infection or a leaking cannula, both of which require immediate intervention.

- **Clinical Response to Medication:** In addition to vital signs, the patient's clinical response to the medication is of vital importance. This may include symptoms such as drowsiness, dizziness, or any other adverse reaction.

- **Adjusting Infusion Based on Response:** Sometimes, it may be necessary to adjust the infusion rate based on the patient's response. For example, if a patient exhibits symptoms of overdose, the infusion may need to be slowed or stopped.

**Considerations for Special Populations**
• **Pediatric Patients:** Children have a relatively smaller blood volume compared to adults and may respond differently to medications. This makes pediatric infusions particularly delicate, requiring special attention in dosing and monitoring.
• **Elderly Patients:** The elderly population also presents unique challenges. With aging, renal and hepatic function may decrease, influencing drug metabolism. This can lead to drug accumulation and potential toxicity if not closely monitored.
• **Patients with Renal or Hepatic Insufficiency:** In these patients, the clearance of many drugs is compromised. As a result, dosages and infusion rates may need adjustment to prevent overdose or toxicity.

## Educating the Patient About Infusion

It is essential for patients to understand the IV therapy they are receiving:

• **Clear Communication:** Nurses should explain the purpose of the infusion, the type of medication, and potential side effects clearly.

• **Post-Infusion Instructions:** Some medications may have long-lasting effects even after the infusion is completed. Patients should be informed of what to expect and when to seek medical assistance.

• **Active Patient Participation:** Encouraging patients to report any unusual sensations or side effects during and after the infusion helps quickly identify potential issues and intervene accordingly.

Overall, while IV pumps and infusion techniques have automated many aspects of care, the human touch and clinical competence of the nurse remain essential. Training, experience, and attention to detail ensure that IV infusions are administered safely and effectively.

## IV Infusion Technology and Equipment

With the advancement of medical technology, equipment used for IV infusions has become increasingly sophisticated:

• **Smart IV Pumps:** These pumps are equipped with software that allows nurses to set dosage limits, offering an additional level of safety. If a specific dose exceeds the set limit, the pump will issue an alert.

• **Infusion Management Systems:** In addition to the pumps themselves, many hospitals now use computer systems to manage and monitor IV infusions throughout the facility. These systems can track dosage, infusion rates, start and end times, and other critical details.

• **Vascular Access Devices:** Various devices are used to access the vascular system, including peripheral catheters, central catheters, and implantable ports. The choice of the device depends on the expected duration of IV therapy, the type of drug administered, and the patient's condition.

**Pharmacokinetics and IV Infusions**

Pharmacokinetics plays a crucial role in IV infusions. This branch of pharmacology studies how drugs are absorbed, distributed, metabolized, and eliminated from the body:

• **Volume of Distribution:** This refers to the extent to which a drug spreads into the body's tissues. A drug with a large volume of distribution might require higher doses to achieve effective therapeutic concentrations in the bloodstream.

• **Elimination Rate:** This is the rate at which a drug is removed from the body. Drugs that are eliminated rapidly might require continuous infusion or frequent dosing to maintain therapeutic levels.

## Risks Associated with IV Infusions

Like all medical procedures, IV infusions are not without risks:

• **Infections:** If aseptic technique is not followed during catheter insertion or infusion preparation, there can be a risk of infection. Hospitals adopt stringent guidelines to minimize this risk.

• **Air Embolism:** This is a rare but potentially fatal complication that occurs when air enters the vascular system through the IV line. Modern pumps have sensors that detect air bubbles and stop the infusion if necessary.

• **Infiltration:** Infiltration occurs when the IV drug exits the blood vessel and spreads into the surrounding tissue. It can cause swelling, pain, and, in some cases, tissue damage.

A profound understanding of all these aspects of IV infusions ensures that patients receive the safest and most effective care possible. And while equipment and techniques may change, the goal remains constant: to provide the patient with the correct dosage of the right medication in the safest manner possible.

## Materials for IV Infusions and Their Specifications

IV infusions require a variety of materials in addition to pumps and catheters, and understanding the nature and specifications of these materials is essential:

• **Infusion Sets:** Infusion sets contain a series of tubes that transport fluid from the IV bag to the patient. Some sets are designed to work with specific pumps, while others can operate by gravity.

• **IV Filters:** These are inserted into the IV line to prevent particles such as debris or drug aggregates from entering the patient's bloodstream. There are different types of filters, each with a specific pore size.

• **IV Bags and Vials:** Medications and infusion fluids are often supplied in plastic bags or glass vials. The choice between the two may depend on the nature of the drug, the duration of the infusion, and facility preferences.

• **Sealing Systems and Connectors:** These small components are essential for maintaining a closed and sterile system. There are needleless connectors that minimize the risk of needlestick injuries and can also reduce the risk of infections.

## Environmental Considerations and Storage

Temperature and light can influence the stability of drugs administered via IV. For example:

• **Light Sensitivity:** Some drugs, such as nitroglycerin and dobutamine, are light-sensitive and require opaque bags or tubing to protect the drug from degradation.

• **Storage Temperatures:** While most IV drugs are stored at room temperature, some, such as certain antibiotics, may require refrigeration until they are prepared for use.

## Infusion Monitoring

IV infusion monitoring goes beyond merely observing the drip. Here are some critical components:

• **Infusion Rates:** The rate at which a drug is infused can directly impact its effectiveness and patient safety. For example, too rapid an infusion of a cardiac drug can cause heart problems.

• **Adverse Reactions:** While IV drugs are often administered because they act quickly and can be precisely dosed, they can also cause adverse reactions. Patient monitoring is essential to identify and manage these reactions.

• **Drug Compatibility:** Not all drugs can be mixed together in an IV solution. Knowledge of incompatibilities can prevent the formation of precipitates or drug degradation.

IV infusion, though common, is both an art and a science that requires in-depth training and continuous education to ensure patient safety and efficacy. Every element, from drug preparation to administration, plays a fundamental role in achieving the best possible outcome.

**Protection Against Contamination and Aseptic Techniques**

Maintaining a sterile environment during IV preparation and infusion is of primary importance:

• **Preparation Environment:** The preparation of IV solutions should take place in a controlled environment, such as a laminar flow hood, ensuring that the surrounding air is free of contaminants.

• **Preparation Techniques:** Using aseptic techniques during the preparation of infusion solutions, such as the use of sterile gloves, masks, and caps, minimizes the risk of microbial contamination.

• **Handling IV Sets:** Connecting and disconnecting infusion sets from the patient should always follow standardized protocols to prevent the entry of pathogens.

**Drug Stability and Reconstitution**

Many drugs are supplied in lyophilized or powder form and require reconstitution before use:

• **Solvents:** The choice of solvent (often saline or water for injectable preparations) can influence the stability and efficacy of the drug. Manufacturer instructions should be followed carefully.

• **Reconstitution Time:** Some drugs must be used shortly after reconstitution, while others can have extended stability if stored properly.

**Calibration and Maintenance of IV Pumps**

Ensuring that IV pumps function correctly is crucial:

• **Regular Calibration:** Like any other precision instrument, IV pumps require regular calibration to ensure that delivered doses are accurate.

• **Cleaning and Maintenance:** Pumps must be cleaned regularly to prevent contamination and should undergo maintenance to ensure optimal performance.

**Biocompatibility of IV Materials**

All materials that come into contact with a patient's drugs or blood must be biocompatible:

• **Raw Materials:** Materials like PVC, polyethylene, and other polymers are commonly used for IV sets and bags. These materials have been chosen for their non-reactive properties with a wide range of solutions.

• **Additives and Plasticizers:** Some materials, like PVC, contain plasticizers that may migrate into the IV solution. Although these materials are generally safe, their migration could alter the drug's properties.

## Osmolality and pH Principles

When it comes to infusion solutions, it is essential to consider osmolality and pH:

• **Osmolality:** Refers to the concentration of solutes in a solution and can influence the movement of fluids between cells and their surrounding environment. An infusion with osmolality significantly different from blood can cause cell lysis or edema.

• **pH:** Most drugs have an optimal pH for stability. Infusing solutions with a pH significantly different from that of blood can cause irritation or tissue damage.

## Conclusion on IV Infusion Calculations

IV infusions represent one of the most frequent and complex procedures in healthcare. Whether it's hydrating a patient, administering vital medications, or providing nutrition, intravenous administration plays a central role in many areas of medical care. A full understanding of the various components and considerations for IV infusion is of paramount importance for patient safety and treatment effectiveness.

First and foremost, a deep knowledge of different infusion systems, such as macro and micro drip sets, and their flow rate specifics is essential. For example, understanding the differences between macro and micro drip sets can directly impact the speed at which a drug or solution is administered.

Furthermore, the biocompatibility of materials used in IV infusions is vital to ensure there are no adverse reactions with drugs or the patient's body. Considerations such as the migration of plasticizers from tubing can have a direct impact on drug safety and efficacy.

The stability of drugs during reconstitution and infusion is another crucial factor. Degradation or alteration of drugs can reduce their effectiveness or even potentially harm the patient.

Lastly, the principles of osmolality and pH must always be kept in mind. Administering a solution with inappropriate osmolality or pH can have serious repercussions on the patient's health, including adverse reactions such as cell lysis or tissue irritation.

In summary, while IV infusions are an essential component of healthcare, they require a level of precision, understanding, and attention to detail that goes far beyond simple dosage calculations.

Patient safety and treatment effectiveness depend on the healthcare provider's competence in correctly understanding and applying these principles and techniques.

## 9. Drug Concentration and Dilutions - How to Prepare and Calculate Diluted Solutions

**Drug Concentration and Dilutions** The concentration of a drug in a solution is a fundamental aspect of healthcare calculations, particularly in pharmacology and nursing. The ability to prepare and calculate diluted solutions correctly can have a direct impact on patient safety and treatment effectiveness.

**Basic Principles of Concentration:** Concentration is generally defined as the amount of solute in a given quantity of solvent or solution. It is often expressed in terms of milligrams per milliliter (mg/ml) or similar units. For example, if a solution contains 500 mg of a drug in 5 ml of liquid, its concentration is 100 mg/ml.

**Types of Concentration:** There are various ways to express concentration, including:

- **Weight/volume percentage (w/v):** Indicates the number of grams of solute in 100 ml of solution. For example, a 5% w/v solution contains 5 grams of solute in 100 ml of solution.

- **Volume/volume percentage (v/v):** Indicates the volume of solute in 100 ml of solution. This mode is commonly used to measure the concentration of liquids in liquids.

**Dilutions:** Dilution refers to the process of reducing the concentration of a solute in a solution, usually by adding more solvent. This practice is often necessary when the desired drug concentration is lower than what is available.

**Calculating Dilutions:** There is a basic formula for calculating dilutions: $C_1 \times V_1 = C_2 \times V_2$, where:

- $C_1$ is the initial concentration of the solute.
- $V_1$ is the initial volume of the solute.
- $C_2$ is the desired final concentration.
- $V_2$ is the final volume after dilution.

Using this formula, healthcare professionals can determine how much solvent to add to achieve the desired final concentration.

**Practical Considerations:** It is essential to ensure that diluted solutions are prepared in a sterile and clean environment to prevent contamination. Additionally, once diluted solutions are prepared, it is important to label them correctly, indicating the new concentration, preparation date, and expiration date.

**Common Examples:** A common example is the dilution of a powdered antibiotic. If a nurse has a 1g vial of antibiotic and needs to prepare a solution with a concentration of 250 mg/ml, they would use the dilution formula to calculate the amount of solvent to add.

In conclusion, understanding drug concentration and dilutions is essential to ensure patient safety and treatment effectiveness. The accurate preparation and calculation of diluted solutions require precision and attention to detail.

**Interactions with Other Drugs:** When discussing drug concentration, it is crucial to consider interactions with other drugs. If a patient is taking multiple medications simultaneously, the concentration of one drug can affect the effectiveness of another. For example, some drugs can accelerate the degradation of others, reducing their effective concentration in the body. This concept is particularly relevant in intensive care units or oncology, where patients may take a combination of drugs.

**Stability of Solutions:** Another important aspect to consider is the stability of the drug in solution. Some drugs, once diluted, can break down or become less effective over time. This means that it is vital to understand not only how to dilute a drug but also for how long that drug will remain stable and effective after dilution. For example, some diluted antibiotics may lose potency if stored for too long.

**Contamination Risks:** Diluting drugs, especially in a hospital setting, also carries risks of contamination. If the dilution process is not carried out in sterile conditions, there is a risk of pathogenic microorganisms contaminating the solution. This risk is particularly high with drugs that are diluted and administered intravenously, where contamination could lead to severe infections.

**Interindividual Variation:** Each individual can metabolize and respond to drugs slightly differently. Factors such as weight, age, gender, health conditions, genetics, and diet can influence how a person absorbs, distributes, metabolizes, and eliminates a drug. Therefore, even with a theoretically correct concentration, additional adjustments may be needed based on the patient's response.

**Legal and Ethical Aspects:** The preparation and administration of diluted drugs also involve legal and ethical responsibilities. If a patient were to suffer harm due to errors in drug dilution or administration, legal complications for healthcare providers or the medical institution may arise.

Every step in the process of drug dilution and administration requires attention, precision, and a deep understanding of both pharmacological principles and the specific needs of the patient.

**Using Appropriate Diluents:** Not all drugs can be diluted with any type of solution. Some drugs require specific diluents to ensure their stability and effectiveness. For example, a lipophilic drug might require an oil-based diluent, while others may need saline or dextrose solutions. Using the wrong diluent can compromise the drug's effectiveness and lead to adverse reactions.

**Dilution Techniques:** Dilution goes beyond merely mixing a drug with a diluent. The technique and the order in which components are mixed can influence the final concentration and drug stability. For example, some drugs may need to be added slowly to the diluent to prevent the formation of bubbles or foam that could interfere with the final concentration.

**Environmental Factors:** Factors like temperature and light can influence the stability of a diluted drug. Some drugs are photosensitive and can degrade when exposed to light. Similarly, temperature can speed up or slow down chemical reactions that affect drug stability. Therefore, it is essential to store diluted drugs under recommended conditions to ensure their effectiveness.

**Final Volume:** The final volume of a diluted solution is a crucial aspect to consider. If the volume is too small, you might end up with a solution that is too concentrated, while excessive volume could result in an overly diluted solution. This is particularly important when dealing with drugs with a narrow therapeutic range, where small variations in concentration can have significant clinical implications.

**Verification and Control:** After dilution, it is good practice to verify the drug's concentration. This can be done through chemical methods or, in some cases, visually. Verification ensures that the prepared solution has the desired concentration and is ready for patient administration.

**Training and Competence:** Drug dilution and administration are procedures that require specific training. Healthcare institutions should ensure that their staff is adequately trained and competent in these procedures, given their importance and the potential consequences of errors.

**Support Systems:** In many healthcare settings, electronic decision support systems are used to assist healthcare professionals in the dilution process. These systems can provide guidelines, calculate the correct concentration based on patient information, and flag any errors or incompatibilities.

In summary, drug concentration and dilutions are critical aspects of clinical practice and require a deep and detailed understanding by healthcare professionals. Patient safety and treatment efficacy largely depend on the correct preparation and administration of drugs.

Understanding drug concentrations and dilutions is crucial to ensure the safety and effectiveness of pharmacological treatment. However, it is not just about mixing a drug with a diluent. There are numerous aspects to consider.

First and foremost, selecting the appropriate diluent is fundamental. Many drugs require specific diluents to ensure their chemical stability and prevent adverse reactions. An error in this step could compromise not only the drug's effectiveness but also patient safety, potentially leading to adverse reactions.

Dilution techniques are equally crucial. The speed, order, and methodology in which components are combined can influence the final concentration of the solution. Proper preparation can prevent complications such as the formation of bubbles or foam that could affect dosing.

Additionally, the storage of diluted drugs in recommended conditions is essential. Light, temperature, and other environmental factors can impact the stability of a drug, altering its properties or accelerating its degradation. This can significantly affect treatment effectiveness. One of the most significant challenges is ensuring that the final concentration of the solution is exact. A solution that is either too concentrated or too diluted can have serious implications for the patient, especially when dealing with drugs with a narrow therapeutic range.

However, even with the best practices and procedures in place, human error always remains a possibility. That's why training and competence are fundamental. Healthcare providers must be adequately trained and equipped with the necessary skills to prepare and administer pharmaceutical solutions safely. Electronic decision support systems, where available, can offer an additional layer of safety, helping prevent errors and ensuring correct dilutions.

In conclusion, the preparation and administration of diluted solutions require a detailed understanding and accurate practice. While technology and guidelines can provide tools and support, healthcare professionals' competence, training, and vigilance underpin every step of this crucial process, ensuring that each patient receives safe and effective treatment.

## 10. Pediatric Dosage Calculation - Specific Dosages for Pediatric Patients

Calculating dosages for pediatric patients is an essential part of nursing and medical care, requiring particular attention and precision. Children are not simply "miniature adults." Their physiology, metabolic capacity, and drug absorption differ from those of adults, making the need for specific and accurate dosages crucial. Here is detailed information on this topic:

**Physiological Differences:** Unlike adults, children have a higher percentage of body water and a lower percentage of fat. This can influence drug distribution in the body. For example, hydrophilic drugs may require higher doses in proportion to body weight in neonates compared to adults.

**Metabolism and Elimination:** The livers and kidneys of neonates and young children are not fully developed, which can affect the rate at which a drug is metabolized and eliminated from the body. This may require different dosages or dosing intervals.

**Absorption:** The pH levels in children's stomachs differ from those in adults, which can affect the absorption of some orally administered drugs.

**Drug Formulation:** Many drugs intended for adults are not suitable for children due to taste, size, or shape. Pediatric pharmacology often requires liquid formulations, which must be dosed accurately using tools like oral syringes or droppers.

**Calculation Methods:** One of the most common methods for calculating pediatric dosages is based on the child's weight. However, there can be a maximum limit for the dosage, regardless of the child's weight. For example, a drug might have a dosage of "5 mg/kg" but with a maximum limit of 200 mg.

**Therapeutic Range:** Many drugs have a narrower therapeutic range in children than in adults. This means that the difference between an effective dose and a toxic dose can be very small. This makes dosage precision even more essential.

**Review of Prescriptions:** Due to the complexity and associated risks of pediatric dosages, it is essential for prescriptions to be reviewed by multiple healthcare professionals, such as pharmacists and physicians, before administration.

In conclusion, calculating pediatric dosages is a challenge that requires knowledge, competence, and attention to detail. Errors in this field can have serious consequences, making in-depth training and constant verification essential. The key is to treat each child as a unique individual, taking into account their specific needs and characteristics, and utilizing all available resources and tools to ensure safe and effective therapy.

Calculating pediatric dosages goes beyond simply converting adult doses based on a child's weight or body surface area. Various aspects require further consideration when administering medications to pediatric patients:

**Organ Maturation:** During a child's growth and development, organs undergo significant physiological changes. The rate at which a neonate or young child can metabolize a drug may differ significantly from that of an adolescent. These metabolic differences can influence the duration and intensity of a drug's effects.

**Adverse Reactions:** Children may respond differently to medications than adults. Some adverse drug reactions may be more common in children, or conversely, some reactions may only manifest in adults. Post-administration monitoring is crucial to detect and manage these reactions promptly.

**Comorbidities:** Some conditions or diseases may be more prevalent in the pediatric population, such as genetic or congenital diseases, which could influence the pharmacokinetics or pharmacodynamics of drugs.

**Treatment Adherence:** Administering medications to children can be complicated by factors like taste, consistency, or the need for regular intervals. These factors can influence treatment adherence, making it essential to seek solutions, such as alternative formulations or administration techniques, that facilitate therapy for the child and their family.

**Emergency Dosing:** In emergency situations, it may be necessary to rapidly administer life-saving drugs. In such cases, healthcare professionals should be well-trained not only to calculate the correct dose quickly but also to administer it safely and effectively.

**Parent or Caregiver Influence:** In many cases, parents or caregivers will be responsible for administering the drug to the child at home. These caregivers must be adequately instructed on the correct dosage, frequency, and possible adverse reactions. They play a crucial role in observing and reporting any anomalies or adverse reactions to the physician.

**Special Formulations:** Often, drugs intended for adults are not available in child-appropriate formulations. This may require the preparation of custom solutions or suspensions at the pharmacy, ensuring that the drug is in the correct concentration and form for the child.

Calculating pediatric dosages, therefore, requires a deep understanding of pediatric pharmacology and the specific needs of children in relation to drugs. It's not just about adapting dosages but taking into account a myriad of factors that can influence the effectiveness and safety of pharmacological therapy in this particular population.

## Pharmacological Management in Pediatric Patients: A Complex Realm

Pharmacological treatment in pediatric patients is an area of growing interest and complexity. While children are often referred to as "miniature adults," the reality is much more intricate. Here are some key considerations:

**Physiological Differences:** Children have different gastric pH levels compared to adults. For instance, neonates have a more neutral gastric pH, which can influence the absorption of certain drugs. Additionally, limited renal function in neonates and young children affects drug excretion.

**Pediatric Pharmacodynamics:** Not only pharmacokinetics but also pharmacodynamics, which pertains to how the body responds to drugs, may vary in children. A drug that produces a specific effect in an adult may not have the same effect in a child, or a different dose may be required to achieve the same result.

**Age and Dosage:** The pediatric age range encompasses a wide span, from neonates to adolescents. Pharmacological needs and responses can vary significantly among these subcategories. For instance, the requirements of premature neonates will differ from those of preschool-aged children or adolescents.

**Nutrition and Metabolism:** Nutritional status can influence drug metabolism. Malnourished children may have reduced levels of certain drug-binding proteins, affecting drug availability in the bloodstream.

**Interactions with Other Drugs and Foods:** Children may be particularly sensitive to drug interactions. Moreover, certain foods can interact with drugs differently in children than in adults.

**Adaptation of Drug Format:** Frequently, drugs are not formulated with children in mind. Tablets may be too large to swallow, or the taste of some solutions may be unpalatable. This necessitates reformulation or the use of vehicles to mask the taste.

**Monitoring and Follow-Up:** Given that children may not effectively communicate side effects or adverse reactions, careful monitoring by caregivers and healthcare professionals is crucial.

**Development and Growth:** The prolonged use of certain drugs can influence children's growth and development. For example, some drugs can affect bone growth or the endocrine system.

**Vaccinations and Medications:** Vaccinations are an essential part of pediatric care. The interaction between prescribed medications and vaccines is another aspect to consider in pediatric pharmacological management.

Pharmacological management in pediatric patients is a discipline that requires specialized attention and training. Healthcare professionals must have an in-depth understanding of the unique challenges presented by this population to ensure the utmost safety and effectiveness of treatment.

## Administering Medications to Pediatric Patients: Art Blended with Science

The administration of medications to pediatric patients is an art that intertwines with science, and the delicacy of this practice cannot be underestimated. While adults can often articulate their symptoms and reactions, children may not be able to do so, making it crucial to understand the nuances of pediatric pharmacology.

Here are key considerations:
**Drug Tolerance:** Children, particularly neonates and infants, may have different drug tolerances compared to adults. This can be attributed to maturation and differences in organ function, such as the liver and kidneys, which play a crucial role in drug metabolism and excretion.

**Routes of Administration:** Traditional drug administration routes, such as oral or intramuscular, may pose challenges in children. For instance, intramuscular injections can be problematic in neonates with limited muscle mass. Alternatively, the transdermal route may be explored, but it also presents challenges, such as greater skin permeability in neonates.

**Drug Formulation:** The availability of suitable pediatric formulations is a major concern. While liquid suspensions may seem an obvious choice for children, aspects like stability, taste, and ease of administration must be carefully considered.

**Storage and Stability:** Certain drugs require specific storage conditions to maintain their efficacy. This can become problematic when drugs need to be reformulated or divided to fit pediatric doses.

**Treatment Adherence:** Adherence is a crucial aspect of pharmacological therapy. In children, resistance to drug administration due to taste, drug form, or fear of injections can be a significant barrier. Strategies to improve adherence may include using flavors to mask unpleasant tastes or employing innovative administration devices.

**Long-Term Effects:** While most drug studies focus on immediate and short-term effects, it is essential to consider the long-term effects of drugs administered during childhood, particularly those given during critical growth and development periods.

**Communication with Parents and Caregivers:** Effective communication with parents and caregivers is fundamental. Clearly explaining the necessity, benefits, and potential risks of a drug can help ensure the child receives the necessary care. Additionally, parents can provide valuable insights into reactions and side effects that may not be immediately apparent to healthcare personnel.

The importance of customizing the therapeutic approach for each child cannot be emphasized enough. What works for one child may not be appropriate for another, requiring a high level of expertise and attention from healthcare professionals. Pediatric pharmacology is not just a matter of scaling doses but rather a complex intersection of science, observation, and care.

## Pediatrics: Tailoring Medication to the Young Patients

Pediatrics, by its nature, encompasses a wide range of age groups, from infancy to preadolescence and adolescence. This age diversity introduces additional challenges in dosage calculations.

**Physiological Development:** Children's enzymatic system, essential for metabolizing drugs, develops over time. For example, a neonate might not have fully developed a certain enzyme, influencing how quickly a drug is metabolized and eliminated. This means that the same drug dose could have very different effects on a neonate, a preschool-age child, and a teenager.

**Growth Factors:** Weight and body surface area are fundamental considerations in pediatric dosage calculations. Since children grow rapidly, these factors can change significantly in a short period, necessitating frequent assessments and dose adjustments.

**Pharmacokinetics and Pharmacodynamics:** Pharmacokinetics (how the body handles a drug) and pharmacodynamics (how a drug acts on the body) can vary significantly in pediatric patients. For example, stomach pH, which can influence drug absorption, varies with age. Drug distribution within the body can also be influenced by factors such as body fat percentage and the maturity of the circulatory system.

**Over-the-Counter (OTC) Medications:** Many parents might think that over-the-counter (OTC) medications are safe for their children. However, many of these drugs have not been adequately tested in pediatric patients. This makes it essential to educate parents about the importance of consulting a healthcare professional before administering any medication to their child.

**Off-Label Drug Use:** Many drugs administered to children are used "off-label." This means that while the drug has been approved for use in adults or for a particular condition, it is used in a way that is not specifically approved. This use requires a deep understanding of the drug and close patient monitoring.

**Pharmacological Interactions:** Just like adults, children can be exposed to multiple drugs simultaneously, leading to potential interactions.

The immaturity of children's enzymatic systems can make these interactions more complex and less predictable.

**Atypical Clinical Presentations:** Children may not present symptoms and signs of overdose or side effects in a typical manner. For example, a drug that causes drowsiness in adults might cause excitement in children. These atypical presentations can make it challenging to identify and manage drug adverse effects.

In conclusion, the practice of calculating doses for pediatric patients goes far beyond simple mathematics. It requires a deep understanding of pediatric physiology and pharmacology, as well as careful observation and communication with patients and their caregivers. The responsibility is immense, but equally significant is the opportunity to make a meaningful difference in a child's life.

## Pediatrics: A Branch of Medicine with Unique Considerations in Pharmacology

Pediatrics, as a branch of medicine dedicated to patients in their formative years, presents a set of peculiarities that influence pharmacological decisions.

**Age-Weight Variability:** In pediatric patients, the weight difference between two children of the same age can be significant. A 2-year-old child may weigh much more or much less than another of the same age due to genetic, nutritional, or health-related factors. This variability can affect the appropriate drug dose.

**Drug Tolerance:** Children, particularly neonates, may have different drug tolerances compared to adults. Some drugs that are well-tolerated in adults may cause adverse effects in children or vice versa.

**Routes of Administration:** The route of drug administration can vary based on the patient's age. For instance, while a teenager may be able to swallow a pill, a neonate or young child may require a liquid form of the drug. The preparation and administration of these pharmaceutical forms require precision to ensure the correct dose is given.

**Organ Maturation:** Organs like the liver and kidneys play a crucial role in drug metabolism and elimination. The maturation of these organs can influence how a child metabolizes and responds to a drug. For example, a drug that is rapidly eliminated from an adult's body may linger longer in a neonate's body due to their immature renal function.

**Central Nervous System Development:** Children's central nervous system is continually evolving. Some drugs can impact this development, leading to potential long-term effects. The prescription of drugs that affect the nervous system, such as those for anxiety or ADHD, must be carefully considered and monitored.

**Environmental and Genetic Factors:** Exposure to specific environmental conditions or genetic predisposition can influence a child's response to a drug. For example, a child exposed to certain chemicals in utero may have a different drug response than an unexposed child.

**Therapy Adherence:** Children, especially older children and adolescents, may have difficulty adhering to the treatment regimen. They may forget to take the medication, refuse it due to taste or side effects, or feel embarrassed about taking a medication in front of their peers. These factors can impact the effectiveness of therapy and require strategies to ensure adherence.

## Pediatrics: The Art and Science of Medication Management

In clinical practice, the pharmacological management of pediatric patients demands not only scientific knowledge but also empathy, understanding, and collaboration with the child and their family. The ability to listen to and communicate effectively with young patients and their caregivers is essential to ensure safe and effective therapy.

**Pediatrics as a Unique Discipline:** As a medical discipline, pediatrics carries the particular responsibility of treating a continuously evolving and growing population. This evolution has direct implications for medication dosages, requiring unparalleled attention and precision. From the previous analysis, several focal points emerge:

1. **Importance of Weight and Growth:** Unlike adults, children's weight varies significantly in relation to their growth. Regular weight assessment is essential to ensure that medication dosages are appropriate. This means that an effective and safe dosage today may not be so in a few months.

2. **Physiological and Metabolic Differences:** Children are not merely "miniature adults." Their physiology and metabolism are unique, with developing organs and age-related metabolic functions. These dynamics influence drug absorption, distribution, metabolism, and elimination.

3. **Treatment Response:** Due to physiological and metabolic differences, children may react to medications differently than adults. This can lead to increased sensitivity to certain side effects or,

conversely, a need for higher doses to achieve the desired effect.

4. **Complexity of Pharmaceutical Preparations:** Children, especially the very young, may have difficulty with certain pharmaceutical forms. This has led to the development of special preparations like syrups, suspensions, or suppositories that need to be carefully calibrated to provide the right dosage.

5. **Treatment Adherence:** Pharmacological therapy in pediatrics is complicated by children's natural resistance to taking medicines, their daily routines, and dependence on parents or caregivers for administration. These challenges require innovative strategies to ensure adherence, such as using flavored preparations or incorporating medication into foods or beverages.

6. **Communication and Education:** Effective communication with parents and, when appropriate, with the child themselves, is crucial. Parents need to be educated on how and when to administer the medication, potential side effects, and what to do in case of a missed dose. Understanding and collaboration among the physician, parents, and the patient are crucial for treatment success.

In conclusion, pediatric dosage calculation is a nuanced and sophisticated discipline that goes well beyond simple weight-based proportionality. It requires a deep understanding of pediatric physiology, pharmacokinetic and pharmacodynamic dynamics, and the unique challenges associated with administering medications to children. However, with the right attention and expertise, it's possible to ensure that every child receives the safest and most effective therapy for their health condition.

**Geriatrics: Tailoring Medication for Aging Patients**

The art of geriatric pharmacology is complex and requires a profound understanding of the unique challenges associated with aging. Elderly patients represent a distinct population with specific needs and vulnerabilities that must be considered when prescribing and administering drugs.

1. **Physiological Changes with Aging:** As individuals age, the body undergoes numerous changes. This includes a decrease in lean muscle mass, an increase in adipose tissue, decreased renal function, and reduced hepatic metabolic capacity. These changes can affect drug absorption, distribution, metabolism, and elimination.

2. **Polypharmacy:** Many elderly patients are on multiple medications concurrently to manage

various chronic conditions. This increases the risk of drug interactions and complications, making regular and comprehensive assessment of therapeutic regimens essential.

3. **Increased Drug Sensitivity:** Due to physiological alterations and concomitant conditions, the elderly may be more sensitive to both therapeutic and adverse effects of many drugs. Consequently, the principle of "start low, go slow" might be appropriate (initiating with a low dose and increasing gradually).

4. **Cognitive and Motor Impairments:** Conditions like cognitive decline, dementia, or motor impairments can influence an elderly individual's ability to take medications correctly. This may require simplified dosing, medication reminders, or special dosage systems.

5. **Pharmaceutical Vehicle Considerations:** Elderly individuals may have difficulty swallowing tablets or capsules. Liquid, chewable, or orally disintegrating formulations may be preferable. However, it's essential to consider taste and palatability, as these factors could influence treatment adherence.

6. **Side Effects and Adverse Reactions:** Due to polypharmacy and physiological changes, the elderly are at high risk for side effects and adverse drug reactions. Regular monitoring and

patient communication are crucial for promptly detecting and managing these events.

7. **Psychosocial Aspects:** Isolation, depression, and other psychosocial factors can affect treatment adherence in elderly patients. Involving the family or caregivers in pharmacological management, when possible, is crucial, along with ensuring a holistic and multidisciplinary approach.

In summary, geriatric pharmacology is not just about dosage; it requires a holistic assessment of the patient, considering both physiological and psychosocial aspects. Healthcare providers must adopt a careful, individualized, and multidimensional approach to ensure that elderly patients receive the most appropriate, safe, and effective therapy for their unique needs.

## Geriatrics: Tailoring Medication for Aging Patients

Geriatrics, as a branch of medicine, focuses on healthcare for the elderly. Understanding the needs of this age group is crucial because they present unique challenges and issues, especially in terms of pharmacology.

**Pharmacological Considerations in Geriatrics:** In the context of geriatric pharmacology, the same pharmaceutical molecule that might be safe and effective in a young adult may not be so in an elderly individual due to various factors. For example, plasma proteins responsible for drug binding tend to decrease with age. This means that drugs that typically bind to plasma proteins may remain unbound in circulation in greater quantities in the elderly, potentially leading to an increase in both therapeutic and adverse effects.

**Renal Function:** Furthermore, renal function plays a pivotal role in geriatric pharmacology. The kidneys are essential for the elimination of many drugs and their metabolites. However, renal function tends to decline with age, even in individuals without renal pathologies. This can lead to drug accumulation and potential toxicity if dosages are not appropriately adjusted.

**Gastrointestinal Barrier:** Elderly individuals may also have an altered gastrointestinal barrier, which can influence drug absorption. Reduced gastric acid secretion, for instance, could impact the absorption of drugs requiring an acidic environment for uptake.

**Central Nervous System (CNS):** Another aspect to consider is the central nervous system (CNS). The elderly are generally more sensitive to the effects of drugs on the CNS, such as sedatives or hypnotics. This can increase the risk of falls, a serious issue in the elderly population. Consequently, drugs like benzodiazepines, first-generation antihistamines, and others that can cause sedation or dizziness must be used cautiously.

**Polypharmacy:** In addition, polypharmacy, the use of multiple medications simultaneously, is common among the elderly. This not only increases the risk of drug-drug interactions but can further complicate the management and understanding of the therapeutic regimen by the patient. For instance, one drug may enhance the effect of another or diminish its effectiveness. This makes close monitoring and regular review of pharmacological therapy essential.

**Socioeconomic Aspects:** Socioeconomic aspects are another area that requires attention when considering geriatric pharmacology. The ability to afford medications, access to adequate medical care, and understanding of medical information are all variables that can influence medication adherence among the elderly. Understanding these factors is crucial to ensure appropriate pharmacological care for the elderly, taking into account their unique needs and challenges.

**Comorbidity Management:** A crucial aspect in the management of medication therapy for the elderly is the attention to comorbid conditions. Often, the geriatric population suffers from multiple conditions concurrently, which can interact with each other and with the various prescribed medications. For example, an elderly individual with diabetes and heart failure may require careful assessment of interactions between antidiabetic and cardiological medications.

**Hepatic Metabolism:** Hepatic metabolism is another element to consider. The liver plays a fundamental role in drug metabolism, and its function may be compromised in the elderly due to chronic illnesses, prior medication use, or simply age. Some drugs require specific hepatic enzymes for metabolism, and the presence or absence of these enzymes can vary among individuals and may change with age. This can influence the speed at which a drug is metabolized and eliminated from the body.

**Cognitive Issues:** Cognitive issues must also be reflected upon. Many elderly individuals may have memory problems or other cognitive impairments, which can make it difficult to remember to take medications, understand instructions, or recognize side effects. Additionally, some drugs can have side effects that interfere with cognitive function, creating additional obstacles.

**Social Aspects:** The social aspect cannot be overlooked. Elderly individuals, especially those living alone or in assisted living facilities, may have limited support networks. This can affect their ability to manage complicated pharmacological regimens. They might not have anyone to help them remember to take medications, notice potential side effects, or obtain prescriptions.

## Medication Administration in Geriatrics: A Complex Landscape

The route of administration is another critical factor. While many drugs are available in oral form, there may be occasions when alternative routes of administration could be more appropriate. For instance, a patient with swallowing difficulties might benefit from a liquid or transdermal form of medication.

**Undesirable Effects and Anticholinergic Effects:** Undesirable drug effects, such as anticholinergic effects, can be particularly problematic in the elderly. Effects like dry mouth, urinary retention, blurred vision, and constipation can not only be uncomfortable but also dangerous. Similarly, orthostatic effects, like dizziness or fainting upon standing, can increase the risk of falls and injuries.

**Personalized Approach:** Lastly, it should be emphasized that given the diversity and individuality of each elderly patient, there is no "one-size-fits-all" approach to pharmacotherapy. The approach must be personalized, based on the specific needs of the patient, taking into account their values, desires, and expectations.

The field of geriatrics, especially when focusing on pharmacotherapy, is vast and full of facets that deserve attention.

**Balancing Benefits and Risks:** Another consideration is the balance between the benefits and risks of drugs. For example, anticoagulants may be useful in preventing thrombosis and strokes in elderly patients with atrial fibrillation, but at the same time, they could increase the risk of bleeding, especially in the presence of other comorbidities or concomitant medications. Therefore, the decision to start an anticoagulant in a geriatric patient must be carefully considered, taking into account the individual risk of thrombosis and bleeding.

**Polypharmacy:** Polypharmacy, the use of numerous medications simultaneously, is a common reality in the elderly population. This presents challenges such as potential drug interactions, an increased risk of side effects, and difficulties with treatment adherence. Regular review of therapies is essential, evaluating the actual necessity of each drug and the possibility of simplifying the therapeutic regimen.

**Therapeutic Adherence:** Similarly, therapeutic adherence can be influenced by visual or manual problems that make it difficult for the elderly to read medication labels or open containers. The availability of adapted delivery devices, such as syringes with large numbers or easy-to-open containers, can help improve adherence and treatment safety.

**Pharmacokinetics and Pharmacodynamics:** Pharmacokinetics, or how the body absorbs, distributes, metabolizes, and eliminates drugs, changes with age. For instance, age-related declines in renal function can affect the clearance of many drugs, necessitating dosage adjustments. Likewise, changes in body composition can influence drug distribution throughout the body.

**Sensitivity to Central Nervous System (CNS) Effects:** Elderly individuals can also be more sensitive to the central nervous system (CNS) effects of drugs, such as sedation, dizziness, or confusion. This can be particularly relevant for drugs like benzodiazepines, antipsychotics, or opioids. Sedation, in particular, can increase the risk of falls, which can have severe consequences in the elderly population.

**Atypical Symptoms:** It should also be noted that atypical symptoms are common in the elderly. For example, a urinary tract infection may not present with the classic symptoms of dysuria or fever but rather with confusion or behavioral changes. Therefore, it is crucial to have a high index of suspicion and a thorough evaluation when assessing an elderly patient with new symptoms or changes in their health status.

**In Conclusion:** Geriatrics, as a medical field, focuses on the specific needs of the elderly population, a demographic group that is continually growing in developed countries. This makes pharmacotherapy in geriatrics a fundamental and complex field of study.

The pharmacokinetic and pharmacodynamic aspects of drugs undergo age-related modifications, which influence treatment responses. The aging process leads to physiological changes, such as reduced renal function, which can slow drug elimination, increasing the risk of drug accumulation and toxicity. Similarly, liver function may decrease, affecting drug metabolism. The percentage of body fat tends to increase, and water to decrease with age, affecting drug distribution. These changes may require dosage adjustments or changes in drug selection.

Another factor to consider is polypharmacy, the concurrent use of multiple drugs by a single individual. This practice is particularly common in the elderly due to the presence of multiple comorbidities. Polypharmacy increases the risk of pharmacological interactions and side effects.

Therefore, a regular review of the medications taken by a geriatric patient is essential to ensure that each medicine is genuinely necessary and that the benefits outweigh the risks.

A thorough assessment of the elderly patient should also consider potential obstacles to proper drug administration. Visual problems, motor difficulties, or cognitive issues may make it difficult for an elderly patient to independently manage their therapy, increasing the risk of errors. The presence of appropriate administration devices and clear labels can help overcome some of these obstacles.

In conclusion, the pharmacological management of geriatric patients requires a profound understanding of age-related physiological changes, an awareness of the challenges posed by polypharmacy, and a holistic assessment of the patient, considering not only their medical conditions but also their social context and abilities. The primary goal remains to ensure the best possible quality of life through the appropriate use of medications and the prevention of potential complications.

## 12. Common Errors in Pharmacology: What Can Go Wrong and How to Prevent Them

The safety of patients is of paramount importance in the field of pharmacology and clinical practice. Despite attention and diligence, errors can occur, many of which are preventable. Here is an overview of common errors in drug administration and strategies to avoid them:

**1. Dosage Errors:** These are among the most common errors and can result from a poor understanding of indications, dose calculation errors, or simple distraction. *Prevention:* Regular training in dosage calculation, the use of electronic tools for calculation, and double-checking doses before administration.

**2. Confusion between Similar Drug Names:** Many drugs have names that sound or are spelled similarly, leading to potential errors. *Prevention:* Proper training on drug nomenclature, clear labeling, and the use of electronic alerts.

**3. Error in Route of Administration:** Administering a drug orally instead of intramuscularly, for example. *Prevention:* Always follow the "five rights" (right patient, right drug, right dose, right time, right route).

**4. Timing Errors:** Administering a drug at the wrong time or forgetting a dose. *Prevention:* Use electronic reminders, checklists, and continuous staff training.

**5. Ignoring Drug Interactions:** Administering drugs that interact harmfully. *Prevention:* Ongoing training, use of updated pharmaceutical databases, and consulting a pharmacist when introducing new medications.

**6. Patient-Related Errors:** For instance, administering a drug to which a patient is allergic. *Prevention:* Maintain an accurate list of patient allergies and verify it before administering any new drug.

**7. Lack of Monitoring:** Some drugs require regular monitoring to ensure they do not cause side effects or toxicity. *Prevention:* Clear monitoring protocols and training on the specific needs of each drug.

**8. Technology-Related Errors:** For example, errors in the programming of infusion pumps. *Prevention:* Adequate training in equipment use, regular checks, and equipment maintenance.

In conclusion, the key to preventing pharmacological errors is a combination of training, attention to detail, effective use of technology, and clear communication among all members of the healthcare team. With the increasing complexity of pharmacotherapy, it is essential to remain vigilant and engage in safe practices to ensure patient well-being.

Pharmacology, like all medical disciplines, is a field where precision and attention to detail are crucial. The complexities of drug administration, combined with the uniqueness of each patient, make this area particularly susceptible to errors, some of which could have serious consequences. In addition to the errors mentioned earlier, there are other common scenarios and variables to consider:

**9. Neglecting Patient's Physical Condition:** A patient's overall health can influence how they will respond to a drug. For example, a patient with compromised renal function may not be able to metabolize or eliminate a drug as expected. *Remedy:* Always consider the patient's physical condition and adjust doses accordingly. This may require blood tests or other diagnostic tests.

**10. Expired or Inadequately Stored Medications:** Medications stored under non-ideal conditions or that have expired may not work as expected and could become toxic. *Remedy:* Always check expiration dates and ensure medications are stored according to the manufacturer's instructions.

**11. Lack of Follow-Up with the Patient:** After the administration of a new drug, some patients may have unexpected reactions or side effects. *Remedy:* Regular follow-up with patients, especially when introducing new medications or adjusting doses, is essential.

**12. Ineffective Communication Between Physicians and Pharmacists:** In some cases, prescriptions may not be clear, or there may be confusion about dosages or the frequency at which a drug should be administered. *Remedy:* Clear and open communication among all healthcare professionals involved in patient care is crucial. The use of electronic tools and electronic prescription systems can also reduce the likelihood of errors.

**13. Labeling Errors:** In some situations, drug labels may be confusing, faded, or even incorrect. *Remedy:* Always check a drug's label before administration and ensure it matches the prescription.

**14. Error in Treatment Duration:** In some cases, a drug may be prescribed for a specific duration but may be discontinued prematurely or extended without a clear medical indication. *Remedy:* Always follow treatment duration guidelines and consult the physician or pharmacist if there are doubts.

**15. Over-the-Counter Medication Misuse:** Many patients take over-the-counter medications alongside their prescribed drugs without informing their healthcare providers. This can lead to potential pharmacological interactions.

*Remedy:* Educate patients about the importance of disclosing all medications they are taking, including over-the-counter drugs, supplements, and herbs.

In the field of pharmacology, attention to detail, clear communication, and patient education are essential to ensure that medications are administered safely and effectively. Understanding the multiple variables involved in drug administration and knowledge of common errors can help healthcare professionals provide optimal care to their patients.

## 16. Prescription Transmission Errors:

Prescriptions are often transmitted electronically or via fax. During this process, misunderstandings or interruptions may occur, leading to errors in the received prescription. *Recommendation:* It is essential to always verify every received prescription with the physician or the patient to ensure accuracy.

## 17. Failure to Review the Patient's Medication List:

Patients often take multiple medications, and failing to regularly review this list could lead to unintended pharmacological interactions. *Recommendation:* The patient's medication list should be reviewed at every visit or at least periodically.

**18. Use of Unclear Abbreviations:** The use of abbreviations in prescriptions or medical notes can lead to confusion or misinterpretations. *Recommendation:* Avoid the use of ambiguous abbreviations and ensure all notes are written clearly and comprehensibly.

**19. Lack of Patient Identity Confirmation:** In crowded settings such as hospitals, it can be easy to administer a drug to the wrong patient if their identity is not verified. *Recommendation:* Always confirm the patient's identity before administering any medication.

**20. Pharmaceutical Form Error:** It is possible for a drug to be administered in the wrong form, for example, a solution instead of a tablet. *Recommendation:* Always carefully read the label and instructions and, in case of doubt, consult the pharmacist.

**21. Lack of Patient Allergy Information:** If a physician or nurse is unaware of a patient's allergies, they might administer a drug that could trigger an allergic reaction. *Recommendation:* Every patient should have an updated record of their allergies, and this record should be consulted before administering any medication.

**22. Error in Dosage Frequency:** A patient might receive a drug too frequently or not frequently enough due to an error in reading the prescription. *Recommendation:* Always follow the instructions for dosing frequency and use reminders or tracking systems to ensure medications are administered as directed. Every error in drug administration has the potential to harm the patient. Therefore, it is essential for healthcare professionals to always be attentive, well-informed, and well-trained to ensure patient safety. Ongoing training, protocol reviews, and the implementation of advanced technologies can help reduce the likelihood of errors.

**23. Inadequate Packaging and Labeling:** Unclear packaging or labeling can lead to confusion among medications. For example, two drugs with similar names or similar packaging could be easily mixed up. *Recommendation:* Always check the drug label and compare it with the prescription before administering.

**24. Ineffective Communication Among Healthcare Staff:** The lack of clear communication between doctors, nurses, and pharmacists can lead to errors. For example, if a drug is changed, and the nurse is not informed, they may administer the wrong medication. *Recommendation:* Promote a culture of open communication where staff feel comfortable asking questions and sharing information.

**25. Improper Use of Technological Tools:** While technology can help prevent errors, it can also cause them if used improperly. For example, an error in the electronic order system could lead to an incorrect prescription. *Recommendation:* Ensure proper training in technology use and have a system for checks and verification.

**26. Errors in Administering Multiple Doses:** Sometimes, a patient may receive more than one dose of the same drug if multiple doctors prescribe the same medication, or if there is inaccurate documentation of administration. *Recommendation:* Use electronic systems to track administered doses and have a protocol for prescription review.

**27. Inaccurate Measurement Due to Defective Tools:** Tools for measuring liquids, such as syringes or dosing cups, could be defective or inaccurate, leading to imprecise doses. *Recommendation:* Regularly check measuring tools and replace them if damaged or inaccurate.

**28. Failure to Check for Drug Interactions:** Patients taking multiple medications are at risk for potentially harmful drug interactions. *Recommendation:* Use software or databases to check for possible drug interactions before administration.

**29. Not Considering the Patient's Diet and Lifestyle:** Some drugs may interact with specific foods or beverages, altering their effectiveness or causing side effects. *Recommendation:* Always inquire about any dietary or food restrictions and consider them when administering medications.

**30. Failing to Consider Patients' Metabolic Conditions:** Some patients may have difficulty metabolizing certain drugs due to conditions like renal or hepatic insufficiency. *Recommendation:* Always check the renal and hepatic function of patients and adjust doses accordingly.

These are just some of the common errors and proposed solutions to avoid them. The key to minimizing errors in drug administration is continuous training, effective communication, and proper use of technology.

**31. Transcription Error:** Transcription errors occur when information is transferred incorrectly from one source to another, such as when a drug prescribed orally is transcribed incorrectly onto the patient's treatment sheet. *Recommendation:* Use electronic prescription systems to minimize manual errors and always perform a double check.

**32. Lack of Knowledge of Contraindications:** Without a clear understanding of a drug's contraindications, there is a risk of prescribing it to patients who might have severe reactions. *Recommendation:* Pharmacists and medical staff should have easy access to updated databases and continuous training on new contraindications.

**33. Inadequate Drug Storage:** Improper storage can degrade a drug, reducing its effectiveness or turning it into a toxic substance. *Recommendation:* Ensure that all drugs are stored as per the manufacturer's instructions and that storage areas are regularly checked for temperature and humidity.

**34. Improper Use of Abbreviations:** Abbreviations can often lead to confusion. For example, "QD" (every day) and "QID" (four times a day) could be easily confused if written unclearly. *Recommendation:* Limit the use of abbreviations and adopt institution-level abbreviation standards.

**35. Symptom-Based Prescribing:** Prescribing drugs solely based on symptoms without a definitive diagnosis can lead to inappropriate and potentially harmful treatments. *Recommendation:* Conduct a thorough patient assessment and use diagnostic tests when necessary to confirm a diagnosis.

**36. Lack of Knowledge of Allergic Reactions:** Without an accurate record of patient allergies, there is a risk of administering drugs that can cause severe allergic reactions. *Recommendation:* Maintain an accurate record of each patient's allergies and check it before each drug administration.

**37. Dose Calculation Error:** This can occur when using the wrong formula or misinterpreting a prescription. *Recommendation:* Use electronic tools or specific calculators to assist in dose calculations and always perform a double check.

**38. Failure to Monitor Side Effects:** Not monitoring patients for side effects can lead to complications and long-term issues. *Recommendation:* Establish post-administration monitoring protocols and educate patients on what to expect and which side effects to report. The list of common errors highlighted the importance of proper training, clear protocols, and effective communication among all healthcare staff. Patient safety should always be the top priority in any healthcare setting.

In conclusion, the list of common errors in drug administration underscores the wide range of challenges healthcare personnel may face in clinical practice. These errors can stem from various factors, including lack of understanding, transcription errors, confusion caused by similar abbreviations, lack of knowledge of patient allergies, and negligence in monitoring drug side effects.

Each of these errors not only represents a potential threat to patient safety but also emphasizes the importance of standardized protocols, verification tools, and ongoing staff training. Regular training, double-checking, the use of modern technology such as electronic prescription systems and updated databases, and the promotion of open communication among healthcare team members are all strategies that can help minimize the possibility of such errors. A patient safety culture should be paramount in every healthcare institution. This means not only identifying and rectifying errors when they occur but also creating an environment in which staff feel empowered to report potential issues and learn from them. Only through understanding and analyzing the root causes of errors can their recurrence be genuinely prevented in the future. Furthermore, it is crucial to educate patients about their prescriptions, potential side effects, and pharmacological interactions. This education will help patients become active partners in their healthcare, enhancing their ability to report any anomalies or adverse reactions, further reducing the risk of medication errors.

In summary, while errors are inevitably part of medical practice due to human nature, with adequate preparation, effective communication, and verification systems in place, the frequency and severity of such errors can be significantly

reduced. The key is to adopt a proactive approach
to error prevention, rather than a reactive one.

## 13. Double-Check Techniques: Ensuring Safety Through Cross-Verification

Double-check techniques are one of the most
effective safety mechanisms used in healthcare,
especially in pharmacology and medical
procedures. These techniques involve ensuring
that at least two healthcare professionals
independently verify a procedure or action before
it is executed. The main objective is to reduce the
likelihood of errors by identifying and correcting
any mistakes before they can harm the patient.

**The Principle Behind Double-Check:** The
premise of double-checking is that if one person
can make a mistake, two people verifying the
same information or procedure can recognize
and rectify that error. This concept is particularly
relevant in high-risk situations, such as
administering high-dose medications, drugs with
similar names, or invasive procedures that can
have serious consequences if done incorrectly.

**Implementing Double-Check:** To ensure that
double-checking is effective, it's essential for each
healthcare professional to perform the

verification independently, without influencing or being influenced by the other. Additionally, both must have a clear understanding of the procedure or action to be verified and have access to the same information and tools.

**Situations Where Double-Check Is Essential:** Some of the situations where double-checking is often used include:

- Administration of highly toxic medications.
- Verifying the correct patient identification before a procedure.
- Checking the proper configuration of complex medical equipment.

**Limits of Double-Check:** Despite the effectiveness of double-checking, there are some limitations. For example, if both professionals are not adequately trained or are subject to distractions or fatigue, they may both fail to recognize an error. Additionally, in some cases, double-checking may be perceived as a burden and may not always be consistently applied.

**Promoting a Double-Check Culture:** It's essential to promote a culture where double-checking is seen as a necessary step to ensure patient safety rather than an additional task. Regular training, well-defined protocols, and awareness of its importance can help ensure that double-checking is applied effectively and consistently.

In conclusion, double-check techniques are an essential tool for reducing errors in the healthcare environment. However, to ensure its effectiveness, it must be implemented correctly and supported by proper training and a clear understanding of its importance.

**Moving Beyond the Basics of Double-Check:**

**Historical Context of Double-Check:** The concept of double-check can be traced back to a time when medicine began to understand the importance of minimizing human error, especially with the introduction of complex treatments and procedures. Initially, it was believed that errors were inevitable and almost "natural," but over time, the need for methods and strategies to contain them became apparent.

**Interaction with Technology:** With the advancement of technology, equipment and software have been introduced to assist healthcare personnel in double-checking. For example, some infusion pumps now require input from two different operators before certain medications can be administered. This ensures that the double-check procedure is always applied.

**The Psychological Factor:** While double-checking is fundamentally a procedure, there is also a significant psychological aspect.

Healthcare professionals are trained not only to perform procedures but also to communicate effectively with each other. Mutual trust is essential, but maintaining a certain level of professional skepticism is also crucial, ensuring that every action is justified and correct.

**The Role of the Environment:** A well-organized and distraction-free environment is crucial for the success of double-checking. For instance, a noisy or chaotic hospital ward can reduce the effectiveness of double-checking. That's why many hospitals are designing specific areas where verifications can be performed with minimal interruptions.

**Challenges in Practice:** While double-checking is theoretically straightforward, it can present challenges in daily practice. Time pressure, staff shortages, and fatigue can influence healthcare professionals' ability to consistently perform a double-check. Additionally, there may be a tendency to "skip" the double-check if one of the professionals is perceived as more experienced or authoritative.

**Adapting to Treatment Diversity:** While some procedures require strict double-checks, others might call for a modified version. For example, for the administration of a common and low-risk medication, a quick verbal confirmation between two nurses might be sufficient, rather than a comprehensive verification.

**Finally, it's essential to emphasize that double-checking, while extremely useful, is just one of many tools available to healthcare personnel to ensure patient safety. It must be integrated into a broader culture of safety and responsibility.**

The importance of double-check techniques in the medical field cannot be stressed enough, and to fully understand their relevance, we can explore further aspects and details of this practice.

**Assessing the Skills of Involved Professionals:** Not all healthcare professionals have the same level of experience or training in specific therapeutic areas. Therefore, pairing two operators with different backgrounds or specializations can provide a more robust cross-verification, with a greater likelihood of detecting potential errors or inaccuracies.

**Double-Check and Personalized Medicine:** With the evolution of personalized medicine, precision in treatment administration becomes even more crucial. Double-checking can play a vital role in ensuring that personalized therapies, which can vary significantly between patients, are administered correctly.

**Digital Tools and Double-Check:** The digital era has introduced various tools that facilitate double-checking. For example, there are applications that allow doctors to input prescriptions, which are then verified by another doctor or pharmacist before approval. These digital tools can also provide real-time alerts if they detect potential drug interactions or inappropriate dosages.

**Research and Studies on Double-Check:** Numerous ongoing research efforts evaluate the effectiveness of double-check techniques in various healthcare settings. These studies often analyze the circumstances in which double-checking prevented potentially severe errors and seek to identify best practices for effective implementation of these controls.

**Training and Simulations:** Regular training is essential to ensure that double-check techniques are applied correctly. Many healthcare institutions use simulations to train staff on how to perform cross-verifications in real-life situations. These simulations also help identify areas for potential improvement.

**Ethical Aspects of Double-Check:** In addition to practical aspects, there are ethical considerations related to double-checking. The primary responsibility of healthcare personnel is the safety and well-being of the patient. The need to ensure safety through cross-verification can, in some cases, conflict with the need to provide care promptly. In such situations, it is crucial for healthcare teams to have clear guidelines on how to balance these imperatives.

**The Future of Double-Check:** While the practice of double-checking will likely remain a fundamental component of medicine for many years to come, we are likely to see further innovations in this field, both through the introduction of new technologies and through research that identifies increasingly effective methods for ensuring patient safety.

The concept of double-check, although widely recognized in the healthcare sector, also has applications in other industries, further underscoring its importance. When we examine double-checking from a broader perspective, we can explore additional details and facets of this practice.

In the aviation industry, for example, double-checking is a fundamental principle. Pilots use checklists for every phase of flight, from engine start-up to landing. These checklists are often reviewed by both pilots in the cockpit, ensuring that each procedure is followed correctly and that nothing is overlooked. This type of double-check is vital for flight safety.

Similarly, in the nuclear industry, double-checking is crucial. Given the potential gravity of errors in this sphere, multiple individuals are often responsible for verifying operations and procedures. This ensures not only that procedures are followed correctly but also that any anomalies or deviations from the norm are detected and addressed before they can become a serious problem.

In finance and accounting, the concept of double-check can be applied in the form of cross-reviews and audits. For example, when processing a complex financial transaction, it is often reviewed by a second set of eyes to ensure its accuracy. This can prevent errors that could have significant financial or legal repercussions.

**Impact on Training and Professional Development:** Double-check techniques can also have an impact on training and professional development. When a new staff member is being trained in a particular procedure or skill, having a second person observe and evaluate can offer a different perspective and provide more comprehensive feedback. This can expedite the learning process and ensure a deeper understanding of the subject or skill in question.

**Project Management and Double-Check:**
In large-scale projects, it is essential to have multiple levels of review and verification to ensure that the project stays on track. Whether it's construction, software development, or any other type of project, the application of double-check techniques can prevent delays, additional costs, and quality issues.

**Psychology and Group Dynamics:**
Psychology and group dynamics also play a role in double-checking. Two individuals may have slightly different perspectives, experiences, and expertise. This diversity can lead to a more comprehensive and balanced view of situations, allowing the identification of problems or challenges that a single individual might not notice.

**Final Note on Competence and Training:**
Finally, it's worth noting that while double-checking is a valuable practice, it does not replace the need for competence and training. Its effectiveness relies on the premise that the people involved are adequately trained and competent in their respective areas.

**The Historical Context of Double-Check:**
The concept of double-check, as a practice, has ancient roots that can be found in various cultures and traditions. For instance, in ancient civilizations, cross-verification was a method

used to ensure accuracy in accounting and transaction recording. In Egypt, scribes often reviewed and compared their own records to ensure they were error-free.

**Medical Context and Double-Check as a Mechanism of Accountability:** In the medical context, double-checking can also be seen as a mechanism of accountability. In situations where an error can have severe repercussions on a patient's health, double-checking serves as an additional layer of safety. For example, during medication administration, a second opinion can help identify potential adverse reactions, drug interactions, or dosage errors.

**Quality Management and Double-Check in ISO Systems:** In terms of quality management, double-checking is often an integral part of ISO systems and quality assurance programs. These regulations establish rigorous protocols to ensure that products and services meet certain standards. Cross-verification, in this context, ensures that non-conformities are identified and resolved before they can negatively affect the final product or the customer.

**Legal Context and Peer Review:** In the legal field, double-checking often takes the form of peer review. Before a legal document is finalized, it may be reviewed by another attorney or expert to ensure its accuracy, completeness, and compliance with existing laws and regulations. This practice protects not only clients but also legal businesses or organizations from potential legal issues.

**Scientific Research and Peer Review:** In scientific research, when a researcher compiles a paper or article for publication, it is standard practice for the work to undergo peer review. Other experts in the field examine the research to assess its validity, accuracy, and relevance. This process helps maintain the integrity of the scientific body of knowledge by ensuring that published information is accurate and reliable.

**Cybersecurity and Double-Check in Code and Updates:** From a cybersecurity perspective, double-checking can manifest in various ways. For instance, before implementing a software update or security patch, it might be common practice for a second technician or expert to review the code or update to ensure it doesn't introduce new vulnerabilities or issues.

**In summary, the practice of double-checking permeates nearly every industry and discipline. It is based on the understanding that human error is inevitable, but through carefully designed systems and protocols, the likelihood of such errors can be significantly reduced.**

**Extending the Concept of Double-Check to Everyday Life:** The concept of double-check, although well-established in many professions, can also be extended to everyday life and personal decisions. Think, for example, of how many times you've sought a second opinion before making an important decision. This instinct to seek confirmation or validation is a reflection of our innate desire to avoid errors and make informed choices.

**Psychological Perspective:** From a psychological perspective, double-checking can also serve as a defense mechanism against confirmation bias, which is the tendency to seek, interpret, and remember information in a way that confirms our pre-existing beliefs. When we seek a second opinion or involve someone else in the decision-making process, we're able to challenge our assumptions and broaden our perspective.

**Educational Context:** In an educational context, double-checking is often incorporated into the learning process as a method to reinforce understanding. Teachers may ask students to review their own work or have it examined by a classmate. This not only promotes accuracy but also teaches students the importance of self-assessment and critical reflection.

**Double-Check in Engineering and Architecture:** Double-check practices have found application in fields such as engineering and architecture. Before the construction of a building or a bridge, for instance, the designs and calculations are often reviewed by a second engineer or architect. This practice ensures that structures are sound, safe, and compliant with current regulations.

**Financial Sector and the Critical Role of Double-Check:** In the financial sector, double-checking is paramount. Banks and other financial institutions employ rigorous control processes to ensure that transactions are accurate and funds are managed correctly. This practice protects not only the institution itself but also customers and ensures the stability and reliability of the financial system.

**Use of Double-Check in Non-Governmental and International Organizations:** Similarly, in non-governmental organizations and international organizations, double-checking is used as a means to ensure transparency and accountability. Before funds are distributed or decisions are made, they are often reviewed by multiple individuals or departments to ensure they align with the organization's mission and vision.

**Limitations and the Need for Proper Training and Culture:** However, it's worth noting that despite its many benefits, double-checking is not infallible. There is always the possibility that both parties make the same mistake or that crucial details are overlooked. Therefore, while double-checking is an excellent tool for reducing the risk of errors, it is crucial to pair it with proper training, robust systems, and a culture of continuous learning and improvement.

**The Intrinsic Value of Double-Check:** Double-check techniques represent an essential tool in professions and procedures that require precision and accuracy, but it's crucial to fully understand their value, limitations, and contexts of application. The intrinsic value of double-checking lies in its ability to provide an additional layer of safety. When two independent individuals or systems reexamine and validate an action or decision, the likelihood of error tends to decrease significantly. This not only ensures the proper execution of a task but can also protect against legal liabilities, ensure adherence to professional standards, and increase the confidence of involved clients or patients.

**Limitations and Context of Application:**
However, there are some key limitations to
consider. First, the double-check technique does
not completely eliminate the risk of error. As
mentioned earlier, both parties may make the
same mistake, or there may be a lack of effective
communication between them. Additionally,
double-checking can be viewed as a burden,
especially if it is not well-implemented or
perceived as excessive or invasive control.
**The Context of Application is Equally
Fundamental:** The context of application is
equally fundamental. While in some situations,
such as in the administration of medication in
the medical field, double-checking is absolutely
essential and can literally save lives, in other
situations, it might be superfluous. The key is to
determine when and how to implement double-
checking based on the associated risks and the
criticality of the activities in question.
**In Conclusion:** In conclusion, while double-
checking represents a powerful risk mitigation
tool, it is imperative to use it judiciously.
Organizations and professionals must carefully
assess where it makes the most sense to
implement this technique, always ensuring
adequate training and promoting a culture of
open communication. Only through thoughtful
and informed application can double-checking

reach its full potential as a bulwark against errors and a guarantor of quality in critical operations.

## 14. Enteral Nutrition Dosage Calculation: Feeding Tubes and Their Requirements.

The calculation of dosages for enteral nutrition is an essential component in the management of patients who require nutritional support through feeding tubes. Enteral nutrition is used when a patient is unable to consume or digest food through the mouth, but their gastrointestinal tract functions properly.

**1. Characteristics of Enteral Nutrition:** Enteral nutrition consists of special blends of liquid nutrients, including proteins, carbohydrates, fats, vitamins, and minerals, necessary to meet an individual's nutritional needs. These blends can vary in terms of calorie density, nutrient composition, and viscosity.

**2. Assessment of Nutritional Needs:** Before commencing enteral nutrition, it is crucial to assess the patient's nutritional needs. This includes determining daily calorie requirements based on factors such as age, weight, physical activity, and the patient's clinical condition. Acute or chronic illnesses can significantly alter nutritional needs.

**3. Types of Feeding Tubes:** There are various types of feeding tubes, such as nasogastric, nasoenteric, gastrostomy, and jejunostomy tubes.

The choice of tube depends on the expected duration of enteral nutrition, the patient's anatomical and clinical condition, and the most suitable insertion site.

**4. Rate and Mode of Infusion:** Once nutritional needs are determined, it is important to decide on the rate and mode of infusion. This can be done continuously using a pump or intermittently by administering a certain amount of nutrition at regular intervals. The choice depends on the patient's gastrointestinal tolerance, the type of tube used, and other clinical considerations.

**5. Monitoring and Adjustment:** Once enteral nutrition has commenced, it is essential to monitor the patient's response. This includes checking for any complications, such as diarrhea, abdominal distension, or regurgitation, and adjusting the rate or composition of nutrition as needed.

**6. Specific Considerations:** Some patients may have specific nutritional needs, such as increased protein intake following trauma or surgery, or restrictions on sodium or fluids due to heart conditions.

In summary, the calculation of dosages for enteral nutrition is a complex process that requires a deep understanding of the patient's nutritional needs and the physiology of enteral feeding. Through accurate assessment, proper planning, and continuous monitoring, it is possible to provide the optimal nutritional support to the patient through feeding tubes.

**Enteral Nutrition Challenges and Considerations:**

Enteral nutrition, while essential for many patients, presents unique challenges that require attention and care. While its primary goal is to provide essential nutrients to those who cannot consume food traditionally, there are multiple variables to consider in its administration.

**Tolerance Assessment:** Healthcare professionals must monitor the patient's tolerance to enteral nutrition. Signs of intolerance may include nausea, vomiting, diarrhea, abdominal distension, and cramps. The presence of these symptoms may indicate the need to modify the formula, infusion rate, or both.

**Medication Compatibility:** Patients with feeding tubes often receive medications through the same tube. This can lead to compatibility issues between nutrition and medications, which could clot or interact with each other. Therefore, it is essential to be aware of and prevent these interactions, possibly by separating the administration of nutrition and medications by at least an hour.

**Infection Prevention:** Another crucial aspect of enteral nutrition is infection prevention. Since the tube provides direct access to the gastrointestinal tract, there is a risk of bacterial contamination. Regular and thorough tube cleaning and proper handling of the nutritional formula are essential.

**Fluid and Electrolyte Balance:** Enteral nutrition can affect the patient's fluid and electrolyte balance. Some formulas may have high sodium content, while others may be more concentrated and require proper dilution. Monitoring serum electrolyte levels and clinical assessment of fluid balance are critical to ensure patient safety.

**Mobility Considerations:** The patient's position can influence tolerance to enteral nutrition. For example, keeping the patient in a semi-upright position can reduce the risk of aspiration. Similarly, encouraging mobility, if possible, can promote better intestinal motility and nutrition tolerance.

**Types of Formulas:** There are various formulas available for enteral nutrition, each with specific compositions in terms of macronutrients, vitamins, minerals, and energy. The choice of the ideal formula should be based on the individual patient's needs, clinical condition, and any dietary restrictions.

**Psychological Aspects:** Finally, one should not underestimate the psychological aspects associated with tube feeding. For many patients, being unable to eat traditionally can have a significant impact on their quality of life and self-esteem. Empathetic communication and psychological support are essential in these cases. Incorporating all these considerations into a patient's enteral nutrition regimen may seem like a daunting task, but with proper training, competence, and attention to detail, it is possible to ensure that every patient receives the best possible care.


**Tube Types and Selection:**
The administration of enteral nutrition can also be influenced by the type of tube used. There are various types of tubes, including nasogastric (NG) tubes, nasoenteric tubes, gastrostomies, and jejunostomies. The choice of the appropriate tube depends on the expected duration of nutrition, the patient's gastrointestinal function, and other clinical considerations.

**Anatomical Location:** The anatomical location of the tube is critical. For instance, a nasogastric tube terminates in the stomach and can be used for short periods. However, if gastric acidity is an issue or there is a risk of aspiration, a nasoenteric tube, which extends into the small intestine, might be preferable. For long-term needs, gastrostomy or jejunostomy tubes are surgically or endoscopically inserted directly into the stomach or intestine.

**Formula Consistency and Viscosity:** The consistency and viscosity of nutritional formulas can vary, and some tubes may be more prone to blockage if used with particularly dense formulas. Therefore, formula selection should be correlated with the tube's diameter and type.

**Infusion Rate:** The infusion rate is another aspect to consider. Too high a rate can cause intolerance, while too low may not meet the patient's nutritional needs. The ideal infusion rate will vary depending on the formula, the patient's ability to tolerate it, and daily calorie requirements.

**Formula Temperature:** The temperature of the formula also plays a role. Administering a formula that is too cold can cause cramps and discomfort, while one that is too hot can alter the nutrient composition. Generally, the formula should be at room temperature to ensure maximum tolerance.

**Hygiene and Cleaning:** Proper cleaning and hygiene during the preparation and administration of nutrition are essential to reduce the risk of infections. The preparation environment should be clean, and hands must be thoroughly washed. Unused formula should be refrigerated and discarded if not used within 24 hours.

**Additives:** Additives may sometimes be necessary to meet specific patient needs. These can include vitamins, minerals, fiber, or medications. However, before adding any supplements to the formula, it is essential to check for compatibility and ensure they do not cause clotting or separation.

**Regular Monitoring:** Finally, regular patient monitoring is fundamental. In addition to checking for signs of intolerance, it is essential to regularly monitor weight, renal function, and electrolytes, among other clinical parameters, to ensure that enteral nutrition is having the desired effect and the patient is receiving all necessary nutrients.

**Tube Material:**

Feeding tubes can also vary in their material composition, including silicones, polyurethanes, and rubbers. The choice of material can influence the tube's lifespan and its resistance to acidic or alkaline solutions. For example, polyurethane tends to be more wear-resistant and less reactive to various medications and solutions, making it ideal for long-term enteral nutrition.

**Complications and Assessment:**

Complications associated with enteral nutrition can range from mild to severe. These may include mechanical issues such as tube displacement or blockage, gastrointestinal problems like nausea, vomiting, diarrhea, constipation, and flatulence, and metabolic issues like dehydration, electrolyte imbalances, and blood glucose alterations. Regular assessment of fluid intake, renal function, and electrolytes can help prevent or manage these complications.

**Proper Nutritional Assessment:**

A correct assessment of the patient's nutritional needs is essential before starting enteral nutrition. This includes estimating calorie requirements, assessing nutritional status through anthropometry and laboratory tests, and considering specific nutritional needs such as proteins, vitamins, and minerals. These assessments help choose the most appropriate formula and personalize the nutritional plan based on individual needs.

**Pharmacological Compatibility:**

In the context of enteral nutrition, the compatibility of medications with nutritional formulas is a critical aspect. Some medications can bind to nutrients or alter the viscosity of the formula, making it difficult to administer through the feeding tube. Additionally, some medications may require absorption in the stomach, while others may need an intestinal environment. Therefore, the choice of the feeding tube and the location of its outlet influence the pharmacokinetics and effectiveness of the drug.

**While enteral nutrition is administered through a feeding tube, oral intake of food and beverages may still be possible and encouraged, depending on the patient's condition. This can help maintain the function and health of the gastrointestinal tract and improve the patient's quality of life. In these cases, enteral nutrition serves as a complement to oral intake, ensuring that nutritional needs are met. Psychosocial Support:** Psychosocial support is also essential for patients with enteral nutrition. Dealing with a feeding tube can be an emotional challenge, influencing self-esteem and body image perception. Offering adequate support, including counseling and education, can help patients adapt to their new situation. **Enteral Nutrition as a Crucial Form of Nutritional Support:** Enteral nutrition, being an essential form of nutritional support for many patients who cannot consume or absorb food through normal digestion, holds a crucial position in the realm of medical care. It involves the use of feeding tubes inserted through various positions, which may include the nose, mouth, or directly into the stomach or intestine.

**Complexity of Enteral Nutrition Dosing Calculation:** The calculation of enteral nutrition doses is complex and must take into account various factors: individual calorie and nutritional needs, underlying medical conditions, medications taken, and potential interactions between these and the nutritional formula, residual digestive function, and potential procedure-related complications.

**Material Selection for Feeding Tubes:** The material used for feeding tubes is selected based on various criteria, including durability, resistance to acidic or alkaline solutions, and biocompatibility. The position and type of feeding tube chosen (e.g., nasogastric, gastrostomy, etc.) can influence how medications and formulas are metabolized and absorbed in the body.

**Complications and Their Management:** Complications can range from mild to severe, and careful and educated management of these tubes, along with a thorough assessment and patient monitoring, is essential to ensure the safety and effectiveness of enteral nutrition. Healthcare providers must be particularly vigilant when administering medications through feeding tubes, as drug-formula interactions can compromise drug availability or alter the composition of the formula.

**Human and Psychosocial Aspects:** Finally, but no less important, are the human and psychosocial aspects of enteral nutrition. Implementing a feeding tube can have a significant impact on body image, self-esteem, and the patient's quality of life. Therefore, it is essential to provide appropriate psychosocial support in addition to clinical management. In summary, enteral nutrition, while being an essential therapeutic modality, requires in-depth understanding, specific training, and a multidisciplinary approach to ensure the best possible outcome for the patient.**

**Clinical Case Studies • Practical Exercises on Real Clinical Scenarios:** Clinical case studies represent an essential component of learning and training in the medical field. Through the analysis of real clinical cases, healthcare professionals can not only refine their diagnostic and therapeutic skills but also develop a deep understanding of the nuances and complexities that characterize medical practice. These scenarios allow for the exploration of a wide range of situations, from the most common to the rarest and most complex pathological conditions.

**Here are some examples of practical exercises on clinical scenarios:**

**1. Case of Heart Failure:** A 68-year-old man presents at the emergency department complaining of dyspnea and swelling in his ankles. He has a history of hypertension and diabetes. How would you proceed with diagnosis and treatment?

**2. Case of Respiratory Infection:** A 4-year-old girl visits her pediatrician with persistent cough, fever, and malaise. She has had contact with other children with similar symptoms at school. What are your diagnostic considerations?

**3. Case of Fracture:** A 30-year-old woman falls while jogging and reports acute pain in her right wrist, which appears swollen and deformed. What steps do you take to manage this situation?

**4. Case of Food Allergy:** A 15-year-old boy eats a protein bar and begins to experience mouth itching, hives, and difficulty breathing. What do you do immediately?

**5. Case of Abdominal Pain:** A 40-year-old woman presents with acute abdominal pain in the lower right quadrant. She also has nausea and has vomited once. What are your diagnostic hypotheses?

These clinical scenarios provide an opportunity to apply theoretical knowledge to practical and real-life situations. During exercises, students can explore various approaches to diagnosis, management, and treatment, receiving feedback from their instructors and peers.

**The Role of Simulation:** It's also important to highlight the role of simulation in this context. Thanks to modern technologies, it's possible to create simulation environments that faithfully reproduce real clinical situations. This offers students and professionals in training the opportunity to practice their skills in a controlled and safe environment.

**Collaborative Learning:** Furthermore, the discussion and analysis of these clinical cases promote collaborative learning, stimulating critical reflection and in-depth understanding. Through this process, healthcare providers can refine their diagnostic and decision-making abilities, preparing to handle a wide range of clinical situations in their daily practice.

**Identifying Recurrent Patterns:** Clinical case studies also serve as a means to identify recurrent patterns in symptoms, diseases, and responses to treatment, providing a basis for developing and updating clinical guidelines and best practices. A detailed analysis of these cases can offer insights into risk factors, comorbidities, pharmacological interactions, and potential barriers to optimal patient care.

**Addressing Uncertainty and Controversy:** Another important aspect of clinical case studies is their ability to highlight areas of uncertainty or controversy in medical practice. This can stimulate further research and clinical studies to resolve these issues and improve the quality of healthcare.

**Personalized Medicine:** In an era where personalized medicine is becoming increasingly relevant, clinical case studies can play a crucial role in emphasizing individual differences in disease presentation and treatment response. This can help doctors develop personalized treatment plans for their patients, taking into account each individual's specific needs and circumstances.

**Ethical Implications:** Finally, clinical case studies can also serve as a platform for discussing the ethical implications of certain clinical interventions or decisions. For example, how do you manage a case where the patient's needs or wishes conflict with established clinical guidelines? Or how do you navigate a situation where there is limited scientific evidence to support a particular clinical decision?

**In summary, through the detailed analysis and discussion of real clinical scenarios, clinical case studies offer healthcare professionals an invaluable means to deepen their understanding of medicine, refine their skills, and contribute to the advancement of medical practice as a whole.**

**Clinical Case-Based Practical Exercises:** Clinical case-based practical exercises are a fundamental element in medical education and ongoing training for healthcare professionals. Through in-depth examination of real cases, doctors, nurses, and other healthcare practitioners can gain a deeper understanding of the nuances and complexities of clinical practice. **Real Clinical Scenarios:** Real clinical scenarios often go beyond the mere text of medical textbooks, presenting unique challenges that can vary depending on the patient's condition, comorbidities, family history, personal preferences, and many other variables. By analyzing these situations, professionals can develop greater empathy for patients, enhance their communication skills, and make more informed clinical decisions. **Interdisciplinary Approach:** For example, a case might involve an elderly patient with multiple chronic conditions, requiring a multidisciplinary approach to care. This might include medication management, physical therapy, nutrition, and psychological assessment. Studying such a case can help healthcare professionals understand how to coordinate care across different specialties and make decisions that consider the patient's overall well-being.

**Another scenario might involve a young patient with ambiguous symptoms that do not align with a clear diagnosis. This could challenge physicians to consider differential diagnoses, explore further diagnostic tests, and communicate effectively with the patient and their family regarding the uncertainty. Addressing Cultural and Socio-Economic Issues:** Moreover, there are cases that could highlight cultural or socio-economic issues. For example, how do you treat a patient with cultural beliefs that may conflict with standard medical recommendations? Or how do you approach a patient who may lack the resources to follow dietary or pharmacological instructions? **Emotional Reflection and Growth:** These real scenarios can also help doctors reflect on their own emotional reactions and biases. After all, medicine is not just about clinical knowledge but also human interaction. Through the reflection and discussion of these cases, professionals can grow both as clinicians and as individuals.

**Legal Aspects:** The legal aspect of medical practice can also emerge in the study of clinical case studies. In an era where medicine is becoming increasingly regulated and subject to litigation, knowing and understanding the various scenarios in which legal issues may arise is crucial. By examining cases that have led to legal action or disputes, professionals can become more aware of risks and best practices to mitigate them.

**A Safe and Supportive Learning Environment:** Finally, it is essential that these practical exercises are conducted in a safe and supportive learning environment. This allows professionals to ask questions, make mistakes, receive feedback, and learn constructively, without the pressure of a real-time clinical environment.

**Clinical Case-Based Learning Approach:** Clinical case-based learning, which involves the study and detailed analysis of real clinical scenarios through practical exercises, represents a milestone in the learning and skill development of healthcare professionals. This educational approach serves to bridge the gap between medical theory traditionally acquired through textbooks and the complex, nuanced reality of clinical practice.

**Key Aspects of this Methodology include:**

1. **Complexity of Clinical Reality:** Real scenarios provide a comprehensive picture of patients, who often present overlapping symptoms, comorbidities, and other variables that can complicate diagnosis and treatment. Learning through these situations helps develop a holistic and multidisciplinary approach to patient care.

2. **Development of Interpersonal Skills:** Clinical case studies allow physicians to refine not only their technical skills but also their communication and empathetic skills, which are fundamental for building trust with patients and their families.

3. **Cultural and Socio-Economic Considerations:** Clinical scenarios often highlight challenges associated with cultural barriers, religious beliefs, or socio-economic limitations, requiring a more adaptive and sensitive approach from the physician.

4. **Reflection and Professional Growth:** Through the discussion and analysis of cases, professionals can identify and overcome their own biases, strengthen their decision-making

ability, and grow both professionally and personally.

5. **Legal and Ethical Aspects:** The examination of clinical cases can also expose professionals to potential legal risks and ethical dilemmas, helping them navigate these complex waters with greater awareness and preparation.

**In conclusion, clinical case-based learning, with its emphasis on experiential real-life learning, offers immeasurable value in medical education. It provides a platform for healthcare professionals to explore, reflect, and learn from concrete situations, ensuring they are not only technically competent but also equipped to handle the interpersonal, cultural, and ethical challenges that inevitably arise in daily clinical practice. When integrated effectively into training programs, this type of learning can lead to more effective, empathetic, and patient-centered healthcare.**

**16. Technological Tools • Applications, Calculators, and Digital Instruments for Dosage Calculations.**

8. The digital revolution has had a significant impact on the field of medicine, offering

healthcare professionals a wide range of technological tools that can assist in their daily functions, improve the accuracy and efficiency of their work, and minimize errors. Focusing specifically on the theme of dosage calculations and pharmaceutical interventions, there are several technological tools that can provide support:

9. **Mobile Dosage Calculation Applications:** There are numerous applications available for both Android and iOS devices that have been designed specifically to assist doctors in dosage calculations. These apps often include features for calculating dosages based on weight, time intervals, and other relevant variables. Many of them are also tailored to specific fields, such as pediatrics or oncology.

10. **Online Medical Calculators:** Dedicated websites offer calculators that can assist in dosage calculations, monitoring renal function, calculating BMI, and many other functions. These online tools are often used to provide a second opinion or to quickly verify calculations.

11. **Electronic Prescription Systems:** These systems are integrated software in hospitals or healthcare facilities that assist doctors in prescribing medications. These systems often include alerts that notify doctors of potential

pharmacological interactions, excessive dosages, or other safety concerns.

12. **Digital Pharmacological Databases:** Accessible through computers or mobile devices, these databases provide up-to-date information about medications, including recommended dosages, side effects, interactions, and other pertinent information. These tools are essential to ensure that therapeutic decisions are based on the most recent and accurate information available.

13. **Simulation Technologies:** Primarily used for educational purposes, these technologies allow healthcare professionals to practice dosage calculations and medication administration in a virtual environment, reducing the risk of errors in real-world practice.

14. **Portable Scanning Devices:** These devices can be used to scan barcodes on medications, ensuring that the right medication is administered to the right patient, at the right time, and in the right dosage.

15. **Artificial Intelligence and Machine Learning:** Although still in its infancy in the medical field, these tools have the potential to revolutionize how doctors make decisions by analyzing vast amounts of data to provide suggestions on dosages, diagnoses, and treatments.

16. In conclusion, while technological tools offer significant advantages in terms of accuracy, efficiency, and safety, it is essential for healthcare professionals to receive proper training in the use of these tools and to maintain a critical approach, always relying on their clinical judgment and experience in addition to the information provided by technology.

17. **Technology has permeated every aspect of modern medicine, and dosage calculations are no exception. Continuing our previous discussion about technological tools available to assist in dosage calculations, it is crucial to emphasize that these tools are functional not only for precision but also for patient safety.**

18. **Integrated Monitoring Systems:** Some medical devices, such as infusion pumps, now come with integrated systems that monitor the amount of medication delivered and can send alerts if there is a deviation from the prescribed dosage. These systems can also connect to electronic patient records for complete traceability.

19. **Professional Feedback Networks:** Some technological platforms encourage doctors to share their experiences and lessons learned regarding dosage calculations. These online

platforms function as forums where professionals can discuss specific cases, share tips, and provide solutions to common challenges.

20.      **Wearables and Telemedicine:** With the advancement of wearable technology, there are now devices that can continuously monitor various patient parameters, such as heart rate, blood pressure, and glucose levels. This data can be used to adjust dosages of certain medications in real-time, especially in patients with chronic conditions.

**22. Virtual Reality Training:** Virtual reality (VR) is becoming a valuable tool in medical training. Through VR simulation, doctors can "practice" dosage calculations and medication administration in a safe environment, allowing them to make mistakes and learn from them without risking real patients.

**23. Predictive Algorithms:** With the evolution of artificial intelligence, algorithms are being developed to predict patients' specific dosage needs. These algorithms use historical data, medical literature, and patient information to make accurate predictions.

**24. User Interface and Design:** While it may seem like a secondary aspect, the user interface design of technological tools plays a crucial role. An intuitive and user-friendly design can significantly reduce errors and increase efficiency, especially in stressful situations.

**25. Updates and Maintenance:**
Technological tools are not static. With advances in research and knowledge, these tools are constantly updated to offer improved features. It is essential for healthcare professionals to be aware of these updates and receive continuous training.

**26. Cybersecurity:** With the increasing digitization, data security becomes vital. Protecting patient information and ensuring that technological tools cannot be compromised are critical aspects.

Finally, it is fundamental to understand that while technological tools offer a wide range of advantages, they do not replace the competence, experience, and judgment of healthcare professionals. Technology should be viewed as a complement, not a substitute, for clinical skills and discernment.

**The evolution of technology in healthcare is rapid, and with the expansion of digital capabilities, the importance of technological tools in dosage calculation and medication administration becomes increasingly evident. When approaching this topic, several key elements need to be considered:**

**Interoperability of Systems:** In an era where information is exchanged at incredible speeds, interoperability between different platforms and software is crucial. For example, a mobile application that assists in dosage calculations should be able to communicate seamlessly with an electronic health record system to ensure that patient information is always up-to-date and accurate. This seamless connection between devices can help prevent errors due to outdated or inaccurate information.

**User Adaptability:** Every healthcare professional has their own working method and level of familiarity with technology. Technological tools should be designed to be intuitive and adaptable to individual needs. Customization of interfaces, notifications, and features can play a vital role in the effectiveness of such tools.

**Real-time Feedback:** One of the most revolutionary aspects of modern technological tools is the ability to provide real-time feedback. For example, a dosage calculation application could immediately alert the user if the entered dose is outside recommended limits, thus helping to prevent potential errors before they occur.

**Integration with Continuous Education:** Education is central in medicine. With the evolution of technology, it is possible that dosage calculation tools also offer educational modules, tutorials, or simulations, helping healthcare professionals to maintain and enhance their skills.

**Multilingual Support:** In a globalized world, healthcare professionals may often need to work in multilingual contexts. Technological tools should, therefore, offer support in various languages, ensuring that information is always comprehensible, regardless of the user's native language.

**Connectivity and Cloud Computing:** The ability to access information from any device and location is fundamental. Cloud-based tools allow healthcare professionals to synchronize data across different devices, ensuring that information is always up-to-date and accessible.

**Peer-to-Peer Assessments and Reviews:** In an era where online reviews are crucial for selecting a product or service, having ratings and feedback from other industry professionals can assist in choosing the most reliable and effective tools.

The combination of these elements, along with the continuous evolution of technology, makes the landscape of technological tools in dosage calculation extremely dynamic. However, it is always important to remember that technology is a tool at the service of healthcare professionals, not the other way around. Patient safety and well-being should always be the top priority. The technological revolution has significantly influenced the healthcare sector, offering innovative solutions aimed at improving safety, efficiency, and accuracy in various areas of practice. Particularly, in the context of dosage calculation, technological tools represent an invaluable resource for healthcare professionals, enabling them to ensure precise dosages, minimize the risk of errors, and prioritize patient safety.

**Interoperability of Systems:** Interoperability among systems is one of the key features of this new wave of digital tools. The ability to integrate and exchange data across different platforms and applications can ensure continuity in patient care and enhance consistency in therapeutic decisions. This integration can also reduce the risk of errors caused by missing or inconsistent information.

**User Adaptability:** Another crucial aspect is the adaptability of tools to the needs of individual healthcare professionals. Customizing interfaces, settings, and functionalities ensures that the tools are intuitive and easy to use, further reducing the likelihood of errors and improving operational efficiency.

**Real-time Feedback:** Real-time feedback, provided by many modern applications, serves as an additional layer of control, highlighting potential issues or inconsistencies before they can translate into clinical errors. This type of immediate feedback not only enhances patient safety but also builds the healthcare professional's confidence in the technology they are using.

**Continuous Education:** Continuous education is a cornerstone in the medical field, and technological tools can function as learning platforms, offering tutorials, simulations, and training modules that keep healthcare professionals updated on the latest best practices.

**Connectivity and Access from Anywhere:** Connectivity and the ability to access information from any location and device offer unprecedented flexibility, allowing professionals to respond promptly to emergencies or access vital data and information as needed.

**Peer-to-Peer Evaluations:** Finally, the value of peer-to-peer assessments cannot be underestimated. Reviews and feedback from colleagues can guide healthcare professionals in selecting the most appropriate tools, ensuring they rely on proven and reliable technologies.

In conclusion, as technology continues to advance and offer innovative solutions, it is essential for healthcare professionals to remain at the heart of the decision-making process, using technological tools as a means to enhance patient care rather than an end in itself. The combination of proper training, real-time feedback, and customized solutions can help ensure that technology is used to its full potential, always prioritizing patient safety and well-being.

**17. Laws and Regulations:** Regulations on medication safety and administration.
The field of medicine, particularly medication administration, is closely regulated by a range of laws and regulations aimed at ensuring patient safety and establishing high standards of clinical practice. Understanding and complying with these laws and regulations are essential for all healthcare professionals involved in prescribing, administering, and monitoring medications.
**Regulatory Sources:** There are many sources of regulation, ranging from national laws to professional codes of conduct and guidelines from organizations. For example, in many countries, there are national regulatory agencies

responsible for drugs and medical devices, such as the FDA in the United States or the EMA in Europe. These agencies are tasked with evaluating and approving new drugs and monitoring drug safety once they are on the market.

**Patient Safety:** At the core of all laws and regulations is patient safety. This includes ensuring that medications are administered in the correct dose, to the right patient, at the right time, and by the right route. Many medication errors can be prevented through control systems and standardized protocols.

**Training and Qualifications:** Laws often establish minimum training and qualification requirements for those who administer medications. This may include the need for licenses, certifications, or ongoing training. These requirements ensure that those administering medications have the necessary skills to do so safely.

**Storage and Disposal:** Regulations often dictate how medications should be stored and disposed of. This may include specific requirements for refrigeration, controlled substances, or the disposal of expired medications.

**Documentation and Recording:** Maintaining accurate records is a fundamental element in medication administration. This helps track which medications were given, in what doses, and when. Additionally, documentation can play a crucial role in the event of legal disputes or investigations.

**Responsibility and Recourse:** Laws also establish healthcare professionals' responsibilities and provide mechanisms for patient recourse in the event of errors or negligence. This includes potential legal actions, investigations, and sanctions.

**Evolution and Updates:** It is important to note that laws and regulations are continuously evolving. New scientific discoveries, changes in the clinical landscape, or adverse events can lead to modifications of existing regulations or the introduction of new ones. Therefore, healthcare professionals must stay updated on the latest changes and ensure compliance with current regulations.

**In conclusion, laws and regulations regarding medication administration play a fundamental role in ensuring the safety and effectiveness of pharmacotherapy. In addition to protecting patients, these regulations also safeguard healthcare professionals by establishing clear guidelines and expectations for clinical practice. Observing these standards is**

**essential for maintaining public trust and ensuring the best possible patient care.**

**Interaction with Other Laws:** Often, laws related to medication administration interact with or overlap with other healthcare-related regulations. For example, patient privacy laws may have implications for how medication-related information is recorded, shared, and stored. Understanding how these laws interact is critical to ensure compliance.

**International Standards:** With the increasing globalization of healthcare, there are many instances where one country's practices and regulations may influence or be influenced by international standards. Organizations like the World Health Organization (WHO) can establish guidelines that, while not binding, often influence national policies.

**Stakeholder Involvement:** In addition to official regulators, many stakeholders play a role in shaping laws and regulations. These can include professional associations, patient groups, drug manufacturers, and other non-governmental organizations. These groups often provide input, conduct research, and influence public opinion on medication-related issues.

**Experimental Medications:** A particularly sensitive area of regulation concerns the use of experimental or unapproved medications. These may be used in clinical trials or under exceptional circumstances, but there are strict regulations governing how they must be administered, monitored, and reported.

**Impact on Research:** Laws can also influence clinical research. For example, requirements for testing new drugs or reporting side effects can affect how studies are conducted and results are reported.

**Education and Compliance:** Ongoing education and professional development are crucial in a field where laws and practices can change rapidly. Healthcare institutions and professional organizations often offer courses, seminars, and other resources to help physicians and healthcare professionals stay informed.

**Audit and Monitoring:** Compliance with laws and regulations is not merely a passive responsibility. Often, there are active audit and monitoring mechanisms in place to ensure that clinical practices adhere to the required standards. This can include internal controls, inspections by external agencies, or reviews by accrediting bodies.

**Consequences of Non-Compliance:** Violating laws and regulations can have serious consequences, both legally and professionally. In addition to potential criminal or civil sanctions, healthcare professionals can face disciplinary actions, loss of licenses or certifications, and damage to their professional reputation.

While laws and regulations may sometimes appear burdensome or complex, it is essential to remember that they represent a fundamental tool for ensuring patients receive safe and effective care. Having a deep understanding of these regulations and actively engaging in their compliance is a fundamental part of being a responsible healthcare professional.

In conclusion, laws and regulations regarding medication safety and administration are crucial to ensure that patients receive safe, effective, and high-quality treatments. These regulations provide a framework within which medical practices must operate and have far-reaching implications for various aspects of healthcare, from clinical research to daily practice. The legislative landscape in this field is influenced by multiple factors. National decisions can be influenced by the standards and recommendations of international organizations, such as the World Health Organization.

However, compliance with these regulations is not just a matter of adhering to minimum requirements. It is a demonstration of a healthcare professional's or institution's commitment to patient safety and excellence in medical practice. Violations of regulations can lead to severe consequences, both legally and professionally. This may include criminal penalties, disciplinary actions, and, in some cases, the revocation of a medical license. Therefore, it is essential for healthcare professionals to be adequately trained and informed about the laws and regulations in effect. Additionally, the interaction and collaboration among various stakeholders in the field of medicine and pharmacology are crucial. These may include professional organizations, patient groups, pharmaceutical companies, and many other entities. Their collaboration and input are essential in shaping regulations that are both practically feasible and optimal for ensuring patient safety. In summary, laws and regulations on medication administration are a key component of the healthcare system. They provide guidance and a framework that, when followed correctly, will ensure that patients receive high-quality care while simultaneously protecting healthcare professionals from potential legal or ethical complications. As in all professions, the key is continuous education, awareness, and a steadfast commitment to professional excellence and ethics.

## 18. Tips for Studying and Memorizing • Techniques and Tricks to Keep Information Fresh.

Studying and memorizing information, especially in a vast and complex field like medicine, can be challenging. Fortunately, there are various strategies based on psychological and neuroscientific principles that can help optimize the learning process. Here are some techniques and tips for keeping information fresh and easily accessible:

**Spaced Repetition:** Instead of reviewing the same topic many times in a single session (cramming), it's more effective to distribute study sessions over time. Spaced repetition helps consolidate information in long-term memory.

**Pomodoro Technique:** This technique involves using 25-minute study intervals (called "pomodoros") followed by 5-minute breaks. After four "pomodoros," take a longer break of 15-30 minutes.

**Visual Association:** Creating a story or mental image related to the information can aid in better retention. The more vivid and unusual the image, the higher the likelihood of remembering it.

**Mnemonics:** These are techniques that use small tricks or verbal devices to memorize lists or complex information.

**Self-Testing:** Quizzing oneself on recently studied material can reinforce memory and help identify areas that need further attention.

**Group Study:** Discussing and teaching information to others can clarify and solidify your understanding.

**Rest and Sleep:** Sleep plays a crucial role in memory consolidation. Sufficient sleep is essential for effective learning.

**Study Environment:** Maintaining a clean, organized, and distraction-free study environment. Listening to light music or white noise can help some people focus.

**Nutrition and Hydration:** Drinking water and consuming nutritious foods can enhance concentration and study efficiency. Avoid excessive caffeine or sugary snacks.

**Physical Exercise:** Regular physical activity can stimulate the brain, improve memory, and concentration.

**Concept Maps:** Creating diagrams or maps that link related concepts can help visualize connections and better understand the information.

**Feynman Technique:** This technique, devised by the renowned physicist Richard Feynman, suggests explaining a concept in simple terms, as if teaching it to a child, to ensure full comprehension.

**Applications and Technology:** Using applications like Anki, Quizlet, or other digital flashcard platforms to review and test your knowledge.

**Breaks and Relaxation:** Taking short breaks and moments of relaxation between study sessions to refresh the mind and body. Remember that not all techniques work the same way for everyone. It is advisable to experiment with different strategies to find the one or ones that work best for you. The key is consistency, dedication, and an active and reflective approach to learning. Over time and with practice, you can refine your study skills and significantly improve your ability to memorize and recall information. Ensuring that learned information remains fresh and accessible requires a multifaceted approach. In addition to the techniques discussed, there are many other methods and suggestions that can be adopted to enhance memory and information retention:

**Multisensory Integration:** Engaging multiple senses during study can improve memory. For example, reading aloud, writing notes by hand, or using vibrant colors for highlighting can help involve more areas of the brain and strengthen memories.

**Incremental Approach:** Instead of attempting to assimilate large amounts of information at once, try to learn a little at a time. This step-by-step approach can make learning less overwhelming and more manageable.

**Real Connections:** Linking new information to something you already know or to personal experiences can create a "bridge" in your memory, making it easier to remember new concepts.

**Strategic Rest:** A short break after learning something new can help the brain consolidate information. This "defragmentation" period can make a significant difference in retention.

**Memory Games and Activities:** Numerous applications and games are designed to train memory. Challenges like crossword puzzles, sudoku, or games like Lumosity can be helpful in keeping the mind agile.

**Storytelling Method:** Creating a story or anecdote based on what you're trying to remember can make the information more interesting and, therefore, more memorable.

**Problem-Based Learning:** This pedagogical approach puts students in the position to solve real-world problems or cases, often in a group setting. It makes learning more applied and relevant.

**Meditation and Mindfulness:** Practices like meditation can enhance concentration, awareness, and memory. Even just a few minutes a day can make a difference.

**Diverse Environments:** Changing your study environment frequently can help reinforce memory. This is because the brain associates information with the surrounding environment, and having different "scenes" can make information more salient.

**Breathing Exercises:** Deep breathing techniques can improve concentration and oxygenation to the brain, facilitating learning.

**Challenges and Goals:** Setting clear, measurable goals and challenging yourself to achieve them can serve as motivation and reinforce your investment in learning.

**Continuous Feedback:** Asking for feedback or conducting regular self-assessments can help identify areas of improvement and ensure you are heading in the right direction.

Always remember that everyone has their own learning style, and what works for one person may not work for another. The key is exploration and experimentation to find the right combination of techniques and methods that work best for you.

## The Path to Effective and Lasting Memory: Strategies for Enhanced Learning and Memorization

The journey toward effective and enduring memory is not linear and varies from person to person. In addition to the methods mentioned earlier, there are additional tactics and strategies that can optimize an individual's ability to remember and apply what they have learned:

**Mind Maps:** This technique, devised by Tony Buzan, is based on creating diagrams that represent ideas, words, and concepts in relation to each other. Creating a mind map can help visualize and structure information in a more digestible format.

**Association:** Associating new information with images, sounds, or familiar concepts can facilitate memorization. For example, if you are trying to remember a complex term, you might associate it with a word or image you already know.

**Method of Loci:** This ancient memorization technique involves associating information with specific places in a familiar route, such as rooms in your house. When you want to recall the information, you mentally "walk" the route and "gather" the information from each location.

**Spaced Repetition:** Studying information at regular intervals, instead of attempting to memorize everything at once (cramming), can significantly improve retention. This technique leverages the so-called "spacing effect."

**Study Groups:** Working with others can offer different perspectives and memorization methods. Explaining a concept to someone else can also help you understand it better and solidify it in memory.

**Quality Sleep:** Sleep plays a crucial role in memory consolidation. Ensuring you get quality sleep and enough rest can have a significant impact on your ability to memorize information.

**Relaxation Techniques:** Reducing stress and anxiety can help improve memory. Practices like yoga, tai chi, or deep breathing can help calm the mind and enhance information retention.

**Nutrition:** A balanced diet that includes foods like nuts, omega-3-rich fish, fruits, and vegetables can support brain function and, consequently, memory.

**Physical Exercise:** Regular physical activity can improve blood circulation in the brain, thus enhancing memory and other cognitive functions.

**Maintain an Open Mindset:** Being curious and having an open mindset can make you more receptive to information. Curiosity is a powerful driver of learning and can make information more engaging and relevant.

**Minimize Distractions:** Finding a quiet study environment free from distractions like television, mobile phones, or background noise can help you focus better on the study material.

**Rituals:** Establishing rituals, such as listening to specific music while studying, can create an association between that music and learning, facilitating memorization.

It is essential to recognize that not all techniques will work for everyone. Customizing your study method and adapting techniques to your individual needs is crucial to maximize the effectiveness of learning.

The art of memorizing and studying effectively is a complex field rooted in both science and individual experience. The ability to retain and retrieve information is not solely based on what is read or heard but also on how that information is processed, organized, and ultimately reviewed.

First and foremost, it is crucial to understand that every individual has their own learning style. Some may benefit from visual methods, while others might find auditory or kinesthetic approaches more useful. Knowing and harnessing your optimal learning style is the first step toward effective memorization.

The study techniques mentioned, such as mind maps, spaced repetition, or association, are not mere strategies to be mechanically adopted but rather tools to integrate into a holistic approach to learning. This means considering not only what you study but also how, when, and where you study.

For instance, research has shown the importance of context in learning. If you study in an environment similar to where you'll later need to recall the information (e.g., an exam), your memory might benefit. Similarly, maintaining consistency in habits, such as the time and place of study, can further solidify the memorization process.

Nutrition and physical activity, often overlooked, play a crucial role in learning. A well-nourished and oxygenated brain functions better, translating into better information retention. Furthermore, sleep, aside from being a physical restorer, is essential for memory consolidation. During sleep, the brain processes and organizes acquired information, making it more easily accessible later.

Finally, while technology offers valuable tools to support learning, it is also one of the primary sources of distraction. This is why it is vital to learn to manage and limit these distractions to ensure productive study sessions.

In conclusion, studying and memorizing effectively is a skill that develops over time and requires deep introspection and adaptability. It's not just about quantity (how many hours you study) but quality. Implementing effective strategies, staying updated on the latest educational research, and, most importantly, adopting a holistic approach to learning can make the difference between forgotten information and firmly anchored long-term memory.

## 19. Assessment Tests: Quiz and Exercises to Evaluate Your Understanding

While study methods are crucial for acquiring knowledge, assessment tests are essential tools to gauge the depth and strength of that knowledge. Taking regular tests can help identify gaps in understanding, reinforce memory, and boost confidence in one's abilities. Let's delve into how assessment tests, specifically quizzes and exercises, can be effectively used in learning.

1. **Types of Tests:** There are various types of tests, each serving a different purpose. Multiple-choice quizzes are excellent for assessing information recognition. Open-ended questions, on the other hand, test the ability to retrieve and articulate information without hints. Practical tests or simulations can evaluate competence in real-life situations.

2. **Immediate Feedback:** One advantage of digital quizzes is the opportunity for immediate feedback. This allows for the identification and immediate correction of any errors, thereby consolidating learning.

3. **Effectiveness of Retrieval:** Retrieval practice, i.e., the attempt to recall information from memory, is one of the most effective study techniques. Quizzes and exercises compel students to retrieve information, strengthening neural connections and making it more likely to remember that information in the future.

4. **Identifying Gaps:** Through tests, students can identify areas of weakness in their knowledge. This allows them to focus on these areas during study sessions, ensuring more comprehensive learning.

5. **Simulating Real Conditions:** Taking quizzes and exercises under conditions similar to those of a real exam can help reduce test anxiety and improve performance when facing an actual assessment.

6. **Continuous Improvement:** In addition to identifying knowledge gaps, assessment tests can also be used as a benchmark to monitor progress over time. Through repeated testing on a topic, one can see how understanding and memory improve, offering motivating feedback.

7. **Encouraging Metacognition:** Metacognition refers to "thinking about learning." Confronting challenging test questions can stimulate reflection on how one learns, which study

strategies are most effective, and how improvement can be achieved in the future.

8. **Diverse Questions:** A good assessment test will feature a variety of questions covering different aspects of the topic. This ensures that understanding is comprehensive and not limited to a particular area.

9. **Online Tools:** There are numerous online platforms that allow students to create, share, and take quizzes on various topics. These tools can be particularly useful for distance learning or independent review.

In conclusion, assessment tests, especially quizzes and exercises, are invaluable tools in the learning process. They not only help strengthen memory and understanding but also provide valuable feedback that can guide future study sessions. When used correctly, they can transform from sources of stress into powerful allies in acquiring and solidifying knowledge.

## The Fundamental Role of Assessment Tests in Education

Assessment tests are crucial in education and training for many reasons. In addition to helping students measure what they have learned, they also provide teachers with insights into how effective their teaching has been. However, beyond these primary objectives,

there is much more to discover about the importance
and effectiveness of assessment tests.

**Deepening and Applying Knowledge:** When
students know they will have to take a test or quiz, they
tend to study more deeply. This is because the prospect
of being tested encourages students not to settle for
superficial understanding but to seek to apply and
connect the learned information. This type of studying
leads to more lasting and meaningful learning.

**Development of Critical Thinking Skills:** Many
tests, especially those with open-ended questions or
case studies, require students to apply their knowledge
in new or complex situations. This can stimulate and
develop critical thinking skills as students must
evaluate, analyze, and synthesize information instead
of relying on simple memorization.

**Promotion of Responsibility:** Knowing that there
will be a test can motivate students to take
responsibility for their own learning. Instead of relying
solely on the teacher or external resources, students
learn to assess their own abilities and recognize where
they need further study or clarification.

**Adaptation to Different Learning Modes:** Tests
can be structured in many different ways: multiple-
choice quizzes, open questions, practical exercises,
simulations, and more. This variety can accommodate
different learning modes of students. While some may

excel in answering written questions, others might demonstrate their understanding better through practical exercises or simulations.

## Strengthening Long-Term Memory:

The practice of information retrieval triggered by tests can enhance long-term memory. Every time information is recalled from memory, the trace of that information in the brain strengthens. So, paradoxically, being tested on something can actually help remember that thing for longer.

## Improving Concentration and Attention:

When students prepare for a test, they tend to focus their attention and concentration on the subject at hand. This can help reduce distraction and enhance the depth of understanding.

## Enhancing Collaborative Learning:

While many tests are individual, the preparation for them can often be a collaborative activity. Students can study together, quiz each other, or discuss complex concepts. This type of collaborative learning can strengthen understanding and offer different perspectives on the same subject.

In summary, while assessment tests are often seen as a means of assigning grades or assessing skills, they have many other valuable functions in education. They offer opportunities for in-depth learning, memory reinforcement, critical thinking development, and much more. And perhaps most importantly, they can give students a clear understanding of where they stand on their learning journey and where they need to go.

## Beyond the Pedagogical Aspects of Assessment Tests

It is equally crucial to observe the various formats and assessment methods, as well as the psychological implications and their role in today's digital world.

### Diversity in Test Formats:

Not all tests are created equal. In addition to traditional multiple-choice quizzes, there are short-answer questions, project-based tests, oral presentations, and practical assessments. Each format has its own set of advantages. For instance, while multiple-choice tests can measure the ability to recognize the correct answer among various options, open-ended questions can assess a student's ability to express themselves and present an argument.

## Psychological Implications of Tests:

Students react differently to tests. While some may find assessments stimulating and motivating, others may find them stressful or anxiety-inducing. This can depend on a range of factors, including previous test experiences, preparation, learning style, and even personality. Recognizing test anxiety and providing resources to help students manage it is crucial.

## The Role of Tests in the Digital World:

With the advent of technology, online tests have become increasingly common. These offer several advantages, including flexibility in terms of timing and location, automated assessment, and immediate feedback. However, they also present challenges, such as ensuring test integrity in an unsupervised environment.

## Continuous Feedback:

Another crucial aspect of tests is feedback. Tests should not only serve as a means to assign a grade but also as a way to provide students with information about their performance. Constructive feedback can help students identify areas where they need improvement and develop strategies to address their weaknesses.

## Adaptive Tests:

In some settings, tests are adaptive, meaning they adjust to the student's level of ability. If a student answers a question correctly, the next question might be more challenging. This can provide a more accurate assessment of the student's abilities.

## The Role of Tests in Continuing Education:

Not only students face tests during their formal educational journey, but many professions require ongoing assessments, such as certification exams or license renewals. These tests ensure professionals keep their skills up to date.

## Integration with Other Tools:

In many modern learning environments, tests are integrated with other tools, such as Learning Management Systems (LMS), digital gradebooks, and personalized learning platforms. This integration can offer a more comprehensive view of student performance and progress.

Indeed, assessment is a complex and evolving field with many facets to consider. When used effectively, assessment tests can be a valuable tool not only for measuring but also for improving learning. However, as with any tool, it is essential to use them carefully and thoughtfully.

**Assessment Tests: A Multifaceted Tool**

Assessment tests are fundamental tools in the educational and professional world. Going beyond mere knowledge measurement, they provide valuable insights into various aspects of learning and skill development.

**Characteristics of Effective Tests:**

Not all tests are effective in measuring what they intend to evaluate. A good assessment should be valid, meaning it measures what it intends to measure. It should also be reliable, producing consistent results over time. Furthermore, tests should be fair, meaning they do not unfairly favor or penalize certain groups of students.

**Types of Assessment:**

In addition to traditional summative assessment, which tends to check knowledge at the end of a module or course, there is formative assessment. Formative assessment takes place during the learning process and aims to provide immediate feedback to students, helping them identify and rectify learning gaps.

## Integration of Technology:

With the advent of digitization, tests can now include multimedia elements such as video, audio, or interactive simulations. These elements can enrich the assessment experience and make tests closer to real or practical situations.

## Adaptive Tests:

As mentioned earlier, some tests are designed to adapt to the student's level of competence. These adaptive tests can be particularly useful in online environments or situations where an efficient and accurate measurement of a student's skills is desired.

## Peer-to-Peer Assessment:

Another approach to assessment involves using peers. In peer-to-peer assessment, students evaluate the work of their peers. This can offer a different perspective and also help students develop critical assessment skills.

## Self-Assessment:

The ability to self-assess is essential for the development of autonomy and metacognition. Asking students to reflect and assess their work can provide valuable insights and help them become more independent learners.

## Challenges in Test Creation:

Creating a fair and valid test can be complicated. Questions must be clear and unambiguous.

Furthermore, it is essential to ensure that the test is free from cultural or linguistic biases that could unfairly penalize some students.

**Ethical Considerations in Assessment:**
Assessment comes with a set of ethical responsibilities. For example, student information must be treated confidentially. Moreover, providing constructive feedback that is helpful and motivating, rather than demoralizing, is crucial.

**Role of Tests in Continuing Education:**
As previously mentioned, tests are not limited to the educational field. Many professions require regular assessments to ensure that professionals maintain and update their skills over time.

In summary, assessment is a complex field with many facets. When used appropriately, it can be an extremely powerful tool to enhance learning and guide teaching.

**Analysis of Data:**
Once a test has been administered, the collected data can be analyzed to identify trends, strengths, and areas for improvement. The analysis can reveal if a particular question was too difficult or too easy or if there were questions that misled students. This data can then be used to improve the test in the future or to modify teaching strategies.

## Immediate Feedback vs. Delayed Feedback:

While some tests provide immediate feedback, allowing students to know their mistakes right away, others delay feedback. The latter choice can be made for various reasons, such as giving students an opportunity to reflect on their answers or to prevent them from sharing questions and answers with others who have yet to take the test.

## Standardized Tests vs. Customized Tests:

While standardized tests are administered to large groups and designed to provide consistent measurement, customized tests are often created by individual teachers or institutions to assess specific learning objectives. The latter can be tailored to reflect the specific curriculum or needs of a particular class.

## Importance of Practice:

Regular exposure to quizzes and tests can help students become more comfortable with the format and develop effective strategies for tackling them. This is particularly true when it comes to high-stakes tests, such as state or certification exams.

## Use of Simulations:

In some fields, such as medicine or engineering, a traditional paper-based test may not be sufficient. Simulations, which replicate real-life situations, can be used to assess students' ability to apply their knowledge in a practical context.

**Open-Ended Tests vs. Multiple-Choice Tests:**

While multiple-choice tests are easier to grade and can cover a broad range of content quickly, open-ended tests allow students to express their thinking in more detail. The latter can provide valuable insights into the depth of a student's understanding.

**Cheating Risk:**

With the advent of technology and easy access to information, the risk of students cheating during tests has increased. This requires more sophisticated assessment methods and anti-cheating solutions to maintain the integrity of the assessment.

**Cultural Considerations:**

It is essential that tests are free from cultural biases. A question that may be clear and straightforward in one culture could be ambiguous or misleading in another.

**Associated Costs:**

The creation, administration, and grading of tests can be costly. This includes not only financial costs but also the time spent by educators and students.

**Balance Between Assessment and Learning:**

Ultimately, it is essential to strike a balance between the time dedicated to assessment and that devoted to actual learning. While assessment is crucial, it should never overshadow the primary goal: learning.

These are just some of the key aspects related to assessment tests. As always, the ultimate goal should be to ensure that assessment supports and enriches the learning process.

**In the broad landscape of assessment techniques, several additional considerations emerge when focusing on optimizing learning and improving the examinee's experience.**

**Adaptive Testing:**

Some tests, especially digital ones, can adapt in real-time to students' responses. If a student answers a series of questions correctly, the test might propose more challenging questions, and vice versa. This type of assessment, called adaptive assessment, aims to precisely identify the student's level of competence, reducing frustration and anxiety.

**Testing Environment:**

The environment in which a test takes place can significantly influence a student's performance. Factors such as lighting, noise levels, temperature, and seating arrangements can affect concentration and the student's well-being. Ensuring that students are physically comfortable can reduce distractions and allow for a more accurate assessment of their abilities.

**Peer-to-Peer Assessment:**
In some contexts, students can be involved in the assessment process by evaluating the work of their peers. This can develop critical skills and enable greater reflection on one's own abilities and those of others.

**Spacing and Interleaving:**
In psychology, the spacing effect suggests that individuals tend to remember information better when their review is spaced over time rather than concentrated in a short period. Introducing quizzes or assessment tests periodically during a course can help consolidate learning.

**Formative vs. Summative Assessment:**
While summative assessment aims to evaluate how much a student has learned at the end of a module or course, formative assessment occurs during the learning process and helps shape and guide ongoing teaching and learning. Both forms of assessment have value, but it is essential to recognize their differences and apply them appropriately.

**Constructive Feedback:**
Beyond simply marking answers, providing constructive feedback can be fundamental for learning. Feedback that explains why an answer is incorrect and how to arrive at the correct answer can help students better understand the material and avoid future mistakes.

**Test Anxiety Prevention:**
Many students experience anxiety when taking tests or exams. Providing resources and strategies to manage this anxiety, such as breathing or visualization techniques, can improve not only the student's well-being but also their performance.

**Technology and Test Integrity:**
As mentioned earlier, technology has made it easier for students to cheat. However, technology can also be used to maintain the integrity of tests. For example, there is software that can monitor students during online tests, ensuring they do not consult external resources.

**Student Involvement in Test Creation:**
Involving students in creating questions for quizzes or tests can be an effective learning strategy. This can help them reflect deeply on the material and identify key areas to focus on. Assessment, in all its forms, remains an essential tool in education. However, to ensure that it effectively serves learning, it is crucial to consider

the wide range of factors and techniques that influence the assessment experience.

## Assessment in Education: Exploring Beyond the Surface

Assessment is a fundamental component of the educational process. It provides feedback to both students and educators, revealing which concepts have been understood and which areas require further attention or reflection. The use of tests and exercises to gauge understanding is a well-established practice in the field of education. However, as we have seen, there is much more beneath the surface of these seemingly simple tools.

## Recognizing Individuality in Assessment

First and foremost, it is essential to recognize that every student is an individual, and traditional assessment methods may not accurately capture the skills and abilities of all. For example, students with test anxiety may not perform at their best in a traditional exam setting but might excel in alternative assessments or more informal situations. This is why diversifying assessment techniques, including peer-to-peer assessment and self-assessment, can provide a more comprehensive and accurate view of students' capabilities.

## The Impact of Technology

Furthermore, technology has revolutionized how we can conduct and analyze assessments. With the rise of digital and online education, we now have access to sophisticated tools that can adapt in real-time, providing questions based on a student's competency level or accurately tracking the areas where students struggle the most. However, these opportunities also bring challenges, such as maintaining test integrity in an online environment.

## The Importance of Feedback

The importance of feedback cannot be understated. In addition to providing an assessment of correct or incorrect answers, detailed and constructive feedback guides future learning. It helps students understand their mistakes, offering them an opportunity to reflect on their thinking and improve.

## Assessment as a Tool for Learning

Finally, assessment is not limited to testing knowledge; it is also a tool for learning itself. The introduction of techniques like spaced repetition can help students consolidate and reinforce long-term memory. Similarly, involving students in test creation can stimulate deeper exploration and reflection on the study material.

In conclusion, while assessment is an essential element of education, it is crucial to carry it out thoughtfully and informatively. Tests and exercises should be viewed not only as a measure of performance but also as a powerful pedagogical resource capable of guiding, informing, and enriching the learning journey of every student.

## 20. Additional Resources for Learning

In a continuously evolving and digitized society, having reliable additional resources is crucial for maintaining or expanding one's knowledge. These resources offer not only in-depth subject matter exploration but also alternative teaching methods that may be more suitable for different learning styles. Let's explore various categories of resources and why they can be essential in the learning journey.

**1. Books:**

- *Advantages:* Detailed exploration, annotative possibilities, offline access.

**2. Websites:**

- *Advantages:* Access to up-to-date information, a wide range of sources, interactivity, and discussion possibilities.

**3. Applications:**

- *Advantages:* Accessibility, interactivity, personalized learning, progress tracking.

**4. Online Courses:**

- *Advantages:* Flexibility, a wide range of topics, access to world-renowned instructors, certificates, and accreditations.

In addition to the mentioned categories, it is worth noting that workshops, seminars, webinars, and conferences are also valuable resources for learning and networking. Professional associations often offer such events as part of their services to members.

In conclusion, in a world where information is just a click away, knowing where to look and how to assess the quality of resources is crucial. Learning extends beyond the classroom; with the right resources, it can happen anywhere and at any time. Therefore, it is fundamental for anyone, whether a student, a professional, or just an enthusiast, to have a set of reliable resources for deepening, verifying, and expanding their knowledge.

## Exploring Emerging Learning Trends and Resources

In addition to traditional learning channels and the discussed digital resources, it's interesting to note how learning is becoming increasingly fluid and integrated into our daily lives. Let's explore some emerging trends and other resources that could prove useful.

- **Podcasts and Videos:** Thanks to the growing popularity of podcasts, we now have the opportunity to learn through listening. Various platforms like Spotify and Apple Podcasts offer a wide range of educational podcasts covering a multitude of topics. Similarly, platforms like YouTube host extensive collections of educational videos and lectures, often created by field experts. These mediums allow for "on-the-go" learning, perhaps during a train ride or while jogging.

**Online Groups and Communities:** Platforms like Reddit, Quora, and other industry-specific forums are excellent places to learn from experts, ask questions, and engage in in-depth discussions. Not only can you access a wide range of opinions and expertise, but you also have the opportunity to contribute to discussions and share your own knowledge.

**Virtual Reality (VR) and Augmented Reality (AR):** VR and AR technology is finding application in education, offering immersive learning experiences. Whether exploring ancient civilizations in VR or using AR to visualize three-dimensional models of cellular structures, these technologies are revolutionizing the way we interact with information.

**Collaborative Platforms:** Tools like Google Docs, Trello, and Slack allow for not only working together but also collaborative learning. Through resource sharing, mutual feedback, and brainstorming, learning becomes a collective experience.

**Digital Libraries:** Even though libraries might seem to be becoming obsolete, they are, in fact, evolving. Many institutions now offer access to extensive digital collections, ranging from e-books to academic journals and historical document archives. This makes research and learning more accessible than ever.

**Game-based Learning:** Game-based learning utilizes gaming mechanics to teach concepts. This approach has proven effective, especially in the education of younger individuals, but it is also finding application in adult education, providing a fun and interactive way to acquire new skills.

**Personal Learning Networks (PLN):** A PLN is a network of individuals you connect with to learn from. This network may include colleagues, mentors, professors, bloggers, and anyone else who can contribute to your professional learning. In summary, with the advancement of technology and the evolution of pedagogy, learning opportunities are becoming increasingly diverse, interactive, and personalized. Access to information has never been easier, but it is crucial to navigate this sea of resources to find those that are truly valuable and relevant.

**The Significance of Additional Resources**: Professional growth and personal enrichment depend not only on formal education but also on the ability to draw from a wide range of resources. Education doesn't end when you leave the classroom; rather, it continues through a series of supplementary resources that can provide further insights, clarifications, and ongoing updates.

**Diversifying Your Sources**: Using different resources ensures a holistic understanding of a topic. For example, while a textbook may provide the basics, a podcast or webinar might present up-to-date information or different perspectives that further enrich understanding. Websites and applications, with their dynamic nature, can provide real-time updates, while traditional publications can offer depth and solidity rarely matched by digital resources.

**Staying Up-to-Date**: With the rapid evolution of science, technology, and professions in general, it's vital to have access to up-to-date resources. This enables professionals to stay at the forefront, ensuring their skills and knowledge are always aligned with the latest discoveries or trends.

**Adaptability to Different Learning Styles**: Not everyone learns the same way. Some may prefer visual content like videos or infographics, while others might benefit from audio lessons or written texts. Having access to a wide range of resources ensures that every individual can find something that suits their preferred learning style.

**Networking and Collaboration**: By participating in courses, seminars, or workshops, you have the opportunity not only to learn but also to establish connections with others in the field. These connections can open doors to future collaborations, idea exchange, or even career opportunities.

**Final Considerations**: In a world where information is abundant and easily accessible, the key is not just knowing where to look but also being able to discern the quality of resources. So, while exploring various additional resources, it's essential to develop a sharp critical sense, evaluating the credibility, accuracy, and relevance of the information provided. Furthermore, dedicating time regularly to update and refine one's skills through these resources is not only beneficial but becomes essential in a rapidly evolving professional and academic environment. In summary, additional resources represent a fundamental component of continuous education, providing the necessary tools to navigate successfully in the ever-evolving landscape of modern knowledge.

**Conclusion: A Journey into the Science and Art of Calculations in the Medical Sciences**

The importance of correctly calculating dosages in medical treatments cannot be emphasized enough. Even a minor error can have serious consequences for patients' health. This book has covered various aspects of this delicate and crucial topic, from the fundamental calculation process to understanding the specificities of certain populations, such as elderly patients.

We began with the basics: Dosage Calculation, exploring the formulas, techniques, and fundamental considerations that are essential for every medical professional.

We then discussed Limits and Recommendations, highlighting the importance of following established guidelines and always staying within recommended limits.

Clinical Cases and Common Errors gave us a practical overview of the real challenges professionals face and ways to prevent them.

We examined the importance of Double-Checking to ensure safety, and how technology, through Technological Tools, can assist in this process.

Legislation and Regulations showed how rules and regulations are essential to ensure that best practices are followed.

To not forget what we've learned, we explored Study and Memorization Tips, and how to Test Your Understanding through quizzes and exercises.

Finally, we emphasized the importance of additional resources, such as Books, Websites, Applications, and Courses. These tools are essential for those who want to delve deeper or stay updated on new research and discoveries.

**Useful Web Resources**:

1. MedCalc - An online resource for medical calculators.
2. Epocrates - A mobile application providing drug information, including dosages.
3. ClinicalKey - A clinical research platform offering access to a wide range of information, including dosage guidelines.
4. SafeMedicationUse - A website dedicated to preventing medication errors.
5. PharmGuide - An online guide for pharmacists and other healthcare professionals.

For those eager to continue their learning journey and further delve into this topic, we recommend consulting national and international medical and pharmaceutical associations, which often offer courses, seminars, and up-to-date publications on the subject.

In conclusion, we hope this book has provided a solid foundation and the necessary resources to ensure that the dosage calculation process is executed with the utmost precision and care. Patient well-being is our top priority, and through knowledge and continuous training, we can ensure we do our best to guarantee it.